HEALTHY LIFESTYLES

Activities and Selected Readings

Fourth Edition

John Scheer
University of Nebraska

Jan Callahan
University of Nebraska

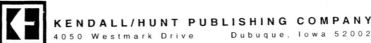
KENDALL/HUNT PUBLISHING COMPANY
4050 Westmark Drive   Dubuque, Iowa 52002

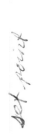

This edition has been printed directly from print-ready copy.

Copyright © 1994, 1996, 2000 by Kendall Hunt Publishing Company

Copyright © 2003 by John K. Scheer and Jan Callahan

ISBN 0-7575-0015-3

Printed in the United States of America
10 9 8 7 6 5

Contents

HEALTHY LIFESTYLES COURSE OUTLINE

DR. JOHN SCHEER, PROFESSOR JAN CALLAHAN

GOALS

The purpose of this course is for class participants to:

1. learn about various risk factors and health behaviors involved in the development of lifestyle-related health problems for college age and adult populations;

2. participate in positive mental and physical health behaviors designed to reduce both short-term and long-term risks; and

3. demonstrate a commitment to a healthy lifestyle by long-term adoption of two or more healthful living behaviors.

Many of the areas of study are of interest to university students who are in the process of forming lifestyle behaviors which can either enhance their health and well-being or lead to premature disease and death. Through the use of a variety of physical and mental health assessments, attention will be focused on health behaviors important to individual participants, and appropriate lifestyle changes will be undertaken.

PHYSICAL HEALTH OBJECTIVES

The course activities and experiences are intended to provide opportunities for class members to accomplish the following cognitive objectives with participation outcomes which enhance physical health. Class participants will:

1. demonstrate an understanding of cardiovascular disease and its relationship to college-age health behaviors, risk factors for disease, and lifestyle behaviors which reduce such risks

2. demonstrate knowledge of the risk factors for cancer, health risks of smoking, and the seven cancer warning signals, and participate in behaviors to reduce cancer risk.

3. demonstrate an understanding of the health benefits and risk reduction of aerobic and strength exercise, and design and participate in an exercise program to achieve such benefits.

4. demonstrate an understanding of, and participation in, nutritional behaviors which meet human needs, reduce chronic disease risks, and lead to achievement and maintenance of healthy body weight.

MENTAL HEALTH OBJECTIVES

Class activities provide students with opportunities to study and participate in behaviors which enhance mental health. Class participants will:

1. demonstrate an understanding of the mental and physical effects of stress, the relationship of stress to immediate and long-term health problems, and participate in stress reduction behaviors designed to reduce such health problems.

2. demonstrate an understanding of the mental and physical health risks of alcohol abuse, and low-risk versus unhealthy consumption patterns.

3. demonstrate an understanding of the mental and physical health risks associated with sex, STDs and AIDS, and risk reduction behaviors.

4. demonstrate an understanding of the guiding principles of self-behavior modification as an aid to behavior change, and participate in a self-designed mental or physical health behavior change program incorporating those principles.

5. study the relationship between self-esteem and mental health, and participate in several behaviors designed to enhance self-esteem.

COURSE MATERIALS

1. Required textbook: Lifetime Physical Fitness and Wellness, by Werner and Sharon Hoeger.
2. Required Course Manual: Healthy Lifestyles: Activities and Selected Readings by John Scheer and Jan Callahan.
3. Blood chemistry profile on announced dates at the University Health Center (2nd Floor east side), 8:00 AM to noon after a 12 to 14 hour fast.

PERFORMANCE EXPECTATIONS

1. Complete all pre and post assessments.
2. Complete blood chemistry profile.
3. Design and participate in 12-week aerobic exercise program.
4. Design and complete 9-week health self-behavior modification contract.
5. Perform satisfactorily on quizzes (≥60% avg.)
6. Perform satisfactorily on the final examination (≥60%).
7. Attend lectures and labs.

COURSE EVALUATION

1. 20%; 9 quizzes
2. 40%; Final Examination
3. 20%; Aerobic exercise program
4. 20%; Behavior modification program

*To pass this course you must pass ALL 4 evaluation factors.

*There will be NO MAKE-UP quizzes.

COURSE FORMAT

The Healthy Lifestyles course includes both class and laboratory activities. During the first week, all class participants will select a time slot for a 50 minute lab. There will be 14 labs beginning the second week of class and continuing through dead week. **Missing more than one lab will cause you to fail this course.**

	Professor:	**Laboratory Director:**
	Dr. John Scheer	Professor Jan Callahan
Office:	250 Mabel Lee Hall	401 Mabel Lee Hall
Phone:	472-1704	472-1715
	jscheer1@unl.edu	jcallahan1@unl.edu

HHPT 100: HEALTHY LIFESTYLES
COURSE SYLLABUS

WEEK	TOPICS	ASSIGNMENTS
Week 1	What is this course all about? What's expected? Exercise: The magic medicine. Video	Text Ch. 1 & 3, Interviews Lab sign-up, 401 MABL
Week 2	Exercise: How much is enough? Max VO$_2$ What will happen if I make it a habit?	Interview task due. Blood chemistry. Text Ch. 4
Week 3	"So You Think You're Going to Live Forever." Can alcohol fit in a healthy lifestyle?	Alcohol reading
Week 4	Nutritional Pre-assessment. What is blood pressure? Stress assessment.	Text Ch. 6 Family History
Week 5	What do my blood chemistry results tell me? Behavior modification topic selection.	Text Ch. 10 Log of Current Behavior
Week 6	How do I design a behavior modification project? "Dying for a Smoke."	Text Ch. 2 Project design
Week 7	Is self-esteem important for behavior modification? "Body Story: Cholesterol Time Bomb."	Text Ch. 5
Week 8	What are my coronary heart disease risks? Dietary fat: How much is too much?	Text Ch. 10
Week 9	Fat, salt, and sugar: What to do? What can I do NOW about osteoporosis?	Text Ch. 8
Week 10	The obesity epidemic: How important is it? What should I weigh? Can I get there with fad diets?	Text Ch. 7 & 9
Week 11	Cancer! Now that's scary! What are my risks? Would I want my children to smoke? What can I do?	Text Ch. 11 & 13
Week 12	How does stress affect me? What are the pathways? How can I deal with stress? Optimize my stress?	Text Ch. 12
Week 13	Sexually Transmitted Diseases: Am I susceptible? STDs: Is a knowledge base important?	Text Ch. 14
Week 14	Alcohol and STDs. Abstinence or monogamy? "It Won't Happen to Me." "Condoms if You Care."	
Week 15	What should I study for the final exam? Final stuff: What kind of lifestyle will serve me best?	Text Ch. 15

HHP 100 LAB

Name _____ Lab/Appt. Time _____ Consultant _____

Lab	Date	Activity	Organization	Comments
1		PreTesting Exercise Prescription	**FULL LAB**	
2		Karvonen Aerobic Log Resistance Training Options	Ind. Appt.	
3		Group Workout (Aerobic) Exercise Logs	**FULL LAB**	
4		Blood Pressure Body Composition Exercise Logs	**Ind. Appt. & Resistance Training Workshop**	
5		Review Wks. 1-4 Goal Setting – Wks. 5-8 Exercise Logs Log of Current Behavior	Ind. Appt.	
6		B-Mod Project Exercise Logs	Ind. Appt.	
7		B-Mod Project Exercise Logs	Ind. Appt.	
8		B-Mod Project Exercise Logs Review Wks. 5-8 Goal Setting – Wks. 9-12	Ind. Appt.	
9		B-Mod Project Exercise Logs	Ind. Appt.	
10		B-Mod Project Exercise Logs	**FULL LAB**	
11		B-Mod Project Exercise Logs	Ind. Appt.	
12		Post Testing B-Mod Summary Exercise Summary	**FULL LAB**	
13		Exit Interviews Evaluations	Ind. Appt.	

Assignments: Blood Chemistry _____, Interview _____, Family History _____
　　　　　　　Grocery Store _____

Quiz Scores (in percentage)

1 _____	6 _____		
2 _____	7 _____		
3 _____	8 _____		
4 _____	9 _____		
5 _____	10 _____		

Quiz Averages (in percentage)

2 _____	7 _____
3 _____	8 _____
4 _____	9 _____
5 _____	10 _____
6 _____	Final _____

PRE LIFESTYLE ASSESSMENT

Following is an anonymous lifestyle assessment which will enable us to describe our classes and see how we're doing from the beginning to the end of the semester. Please be as accurate as possible with your responses.

Below, circle one response in each category which best describes your behavioral pattern as it is now.

STRESS

subscore _____−2_____

- 0   I rarely feel stressed out.
- -1   I sometimes feel stressed out, but I handle it well by exercising, talking, or relaxing.
- -2   I feel stressed out 1-2 days per week, and I could handle it better.
- -3   I feel stressed out 3-4 days per week, and I could handle it better.
- -4   I feel stressed out 5-6 days per week, and I could handle it better.
- -5   I feel stressed every day, and I could handle it better.

ALCOHOL

subscore _____0_____

- 0   I drink no more than 1 drink per hour, 2 drinks per day, and 4 days per week.
- -1   I drink 9-15 drinks per week (-3 if in 1 or 2 days).
- -2   I drink 16-20 drinks per week (-4 if in 1, 2, or 3 days).
- -3   I drink 21-25 drinks per week (-5 if in 1 to 4 days).
- -4   I drink 26-30 drinks per week (-5 if in 1 to 4 days).
- -5   I drink more than 30 drinks per week.

FITNESS

subscore_____−4_____

- 0   I exercise 4 or more times per week for 30 or more minutes of continuous aerobic exercise.
- -1   I exercise 3 times per week for 25 or more minutes nonstop.
- -2   I exercise 3 times per week for 20 minutes nonstop.
- -3   I exercise 2 times per week for 20 or more minutes nonstop.
- -4   I exercise 2-3 times per week for 15 minutes nonstop.
- -5   I never exercise, or I only exercise once per week.

NUTRITION

subscore _____ 0

0   I eat a balanced diet daily which includes: (a) the 5 food groups, (b) plenty of fruits, vegetables, whole grains and fiber, (c) limited fat, and (d) limited sugar.

-1   I usually eat a balanced diet as described above.

-2   I usually eat a variety of foods and concern myself with some, but not all, of the specifics described above.

-3   I sometimes eat a variety of foods and concern myself with 1 or 2 of the specifics described above.

-4   I eat whatever is available.

-5   The majority of what I eat is highly processed food and/or is high in fat, sugar, and/or salt.

TOBACCO

subscore _____ 0

0   I never smoke cigarettes, pipes, or cigars, or chew tobacco; and I limit my exposure to secondhand smoke.

-1   I never smoke or chew tobacco, but I am sometimes exposed to secondhand smoke.

-2   I never smoke or chew tobacco, but I am frequently (several hours per day or more) exposed to secondhand smoke.

-3   I smoke or chew tobacco occasionally.

-4   I smoke less than a pack of cigarettes per day or I chew tobacco regularly.

-5   I smoke a pack or more per day.

Below, circle a score for each of the 4 areas and total your scores for the Safety Subscore.

SAFETY

subscore _____ 0/0/0/0

1.   0   I never drive after drinking or ride with someone who has.
     -5   I sometimes drink and drive or ride with someone who has.

2.   0   I always wear a seatbelt in a motor vehicle.
     -3   I usually, but not always, wear a seatbelt.
     -5   I rarely or never wear a seatbelt.

3.   0   I never use illegal drugs (not including alcohol).
     -5   I sometimes use illegal drugs.

4.   0   I abstain from sex, or I have a monogamous relationship with someone I am certain is free of STDs or HIV, or I always practice safer sex.
     -5   I sometimes do not practice safer sex and/or I am uncertain about the sexual history of my partner(s).

TOTAL PRE LIFESTYLE ASSESSMENT SCORE = _____ −6

POST LIFESTYLE ASSESSMENT

Following is an anonymous lifestyle assessment which will enable us to describe our classes and see how we're doing from the beginning to the end of the semester. Please be as accurate as possible with your responses.

Below, circle one response in each category which best describes your behavioral pattern at the end of the semester. Staple this form to your pre-assessment and place them in the anonymous envelope at lab check-out during Dead Week.

STRESS

subscore _____

0	I rarely feel stressed out.
-1	I sometimes feel stressed out, but I handle it well by exercising, talking, or relaxing.
-2	I feel stressed out 1-2 days per week, and I could handle it better.
-3	I feel stressed out 3-4 days per week, and I could handle it better.
-4	I feel stressed out 5-6 days per week, and I could handle it better.
-5	I feel stressed every day, and I could handle it better.

ALCOHOL

subscore _____

0	I drink no more than 1 drink per hour, 2 drinks per day, and 4 days per week.
-1	I drink 9-15 drinks per week (-3 if in 1 or 2 days).
-2	I drink 16-20 drinks per week (-4 if in 1, 2, or 3 days).
-3	I drink 21-25 drinks per week (-5 if in 1 to 4 days).
-4	I drink 26-30 drinks per week (-5 if in 1 to 4 days).
-5	I drink more than 30 drinks per week.

FITNESS

subscore_____

0	I exercise 4 or more times per week for 30 or more minutes of continuous aerobic exercise.
-1	I exercise 3 times per week for 25 or more minutes nonstop.
-2	I exercise 3 times per week for 20 minutes nonstop.
-3	I exercise 2 times per week for 20 or more minutes nonstop.
-4	I exercise 2-3 times per week for 15 minutes nonstop.
-5	I never exercise, or I only exercise once per week.

NUTRITION

subscore _____

0   I eat a balanced diet daily which includes: (a) the 5 food groups, (b) plenty of fruits, vegetables, whole grains and fiber, (c) limited fat, and (d) limited sugar.

-1   I usually eat a balanced diet as described above.

-2   I usually eat a variety of foods and concern myself with some, but not all, of the specifics described above.

-3   I sometimes eat a variety of foods and concern myself with 1 or 2 of the specifics described above.

-4   I eat whatever is available.

-5   The majority of what I eat is highly processed food and/or is high in fat, sugar, and/or salt.

TOBACCO

subscore _____

0   I never smoke cigarettes, pipes, or cigars, or chew tobacco; and I limit my exposure to secondhand smoke.

-1   I never smoke or chew tobacco, but I am sometimes exposed to secondhand smoke.

-2   I never smoke or chew tobacco, but I am frequently (several hours per day or more) exposed to secondhand smoke.

-3   I smoke or chew tobacco occasionally.

-4   I smoke less than a pack of cigarettes per day or I chew tobacco regularly.

-5   I smoke a pack or more per day.

Below, circle a score for each of the 4 areas and total your scores for the Safety Subscore.

SAFETY

subscore _____

1.   0   I never drive after drinking or ride with someone who has.
      -5   I sometimes drink and drive or ride with someone who has.

2.   0   I always wear a seatbelt in a motor vehicle.
      -3   I usually, but not always, wear a seatbelt.
      -5   I rarely or never wear a seatbelt.

3.   0   I never use illegal drugs (not including alcohol).
      -5   I sometimes use illegal drugs.

4.   0   I abstain from sex, or I have a monogamous relationship with someone I am certain is free of STDs or HIV, or I always practice safer sex.
      -5   I sometimes do not practice safer sex and/or I am uncertain about the sexual history of my partner(s).

TOTAL POST LIFESTYLE ASSESSMENT SCORE = _____

HHP 100 Lab
Student Data/course Participation Form

Name ___Shiloh Hooker___ Age __22__ Sex __F__ Soc/Sec# _____

Email Address ___gregsgirl 5205___

Campus Address _____ Campus Phone _____

Permanent Address _____ Home Phone _484-6840_

City, State & Zip _____ Work Phone _____

Birth date __9/8__ Major _____ Year in School FO SO JR SR GR (5th)

  HHP 100 contains a rigorous exercise dimension. We encourage you to be fully aware of your present physical condition before contracting your aerobic exercise program.

  When signing this form you agree to accept the responsibility for your health and safety, and you also agree to keep the Healthy Lifestyles Lab Staff informed on any physical limitations and/or changes that might influence your reaction to your exercise prescription.

***Please visit with the Lab supervisor if you are 35 or older, have one or more major risk factors, or you answered Yes to any question on PAR Q.

___Shiloh Hooker___   ___9-11-06___
(Signature)   (Date)

PHYSICAL ASSESSMENTS/CURRENT PROGRAMS

Client _____

	PRE	POST	LIFETIME GOAL
Step Test	15 Sec HR _____ 60 Sec HR _____ VO₂ _____	15 Sec HR _____ 60 Sec HR _____ VO₂ _____	
Sit/Reach			
Blood Pressure			
Body Composition	____ ____ ____ Sum _____ % _____	____ ____ ____ Sum _____ % _____	

Circle the items that describe you

General attitudes towards exercising:
1. I love it.
2. I hate it.
3. I can take it or leave it.
4. I know it is good for me but I'm not disciplined about doing it.
5. I need to exercise several days each week to feel good about myself.

Present habits related to aerobic exercise:
1. I do not do any aerobic exercise.
2. I play intramural team sports or pick up basketball or soccer at least 2 x a week.
3. I do some aerobic activity at least 2 x a week.
4. I schedule 3-5 aerobic activities of 30-60 minutes in each week.

Present habits related to resistance training:
1. I do not do any resistance training.
2. I do specific exercises such as pushups and abdominal work 2-3 x a week.
3. I do a few upper body exercises 2 x a week.
4. I schedule 2-4 full body workouts in each week.

Present habits related to flexibility:
1. I do not do any flexibility work.
2. I do a few minutes of stretching after I work out.
3. I include some form of yoga or tai chi in my schedule at least 2 x a week.
4. I stretch for at least 10 minutes after every workout.

If you are an UNL athlete and/or an athlete preparing for an endurance competition, please identify your sport.

Resting Heart Rate

Your Resting Heart Rate (RHR) is a good indicator of your cardiorespiratory fitness. To take your RHR, use the radial (wrist) or carotid (neck) artery and count your pulse for a **FULL 60 SECONDS**, starting with ZERO. Do not use your thumb to take your pulse because it also has a pulse and will result in an inaccurate reading. **Take your RHR twice every day and average the two together.** At the end of the week average the 7 RHRs. The best time to take a RHR is in the morning before you get out of bed. If you are unable to get a reading in the morning, you can take a reading in the evening when you have been inactive for 30 minutes or longer (ex. After studying, reading, or lying down).

Week #1	Mon	Tue	Wed	Thurs	Fri	Sat	Sun	Average
RHR								
AM/PM								
Time of Day								
Place								

Week #2	Mon	Tue	Wed	Thurs	Fri	Sat	Sun	Average
RHR								
AM/PM								
Time of Day								
Place								

Week #3	Mon	Tue	Wed	Thurs	Fri	Sat	Sun	Average
RHR								
AM/PM								
Time of Day								
Place								

Week #4	Mon	Tue	Wed	Thurs	Fri	Sat	Sun	Average
RHR								
AM/PM								
Time of Day								
Place								

RHR _____

EHR @ 50% ___|___ @ 60% ___|___ @ 70% ___|___ @ 75% ___|___ @ 80% ___|___ @ 85% ___|___.

GOALS:

Week	Aerobic				Resistance Training				
	Activity	Intensity	Duration	Frequency	Type	Frequency	#Exercises	Sets	Reps
1									
2									
3									
4									

Summary:

RHR _____

CLIENT _____ Exercise Classification _____ Consultant _____

AEROBIC EXERCISE LOG

Week # _____   Intensity _____ - _____   Duration _____ - _____   Frequency _____ - _____

DAY/DATE							
WARM UP ACTIVITY							
MINUTES HR							
WORK OUT ACTIVITY							
HR@1/2 WAY HR@ END **TOTAL MINUTES**							
COOL DOWN ACTIVITY							
# OF MINUTES TO GET HR DOWN TO 100							
STRETCHING #SECONDS HELD EACH STRETCH							
TOTAL MINUTES							
THOUGHTS (ABOUT YOUR WO) - BEFORE							
- DURING							
- AFTER							

AEROBIC EXERCISE LOG Week # _____ Intensity _____ - _____ Duration _____ - _____ Frequency _____ - _____

DAY/DATE							
WARM UP ACTIVITY							
MINUTES HR	___ ___	___ ___	___ ___	___ ___	___ ___	___ ___	
WORK OUT ACTIVITY							
HR@1/2 WAY HR@ END **TOTAL MINUTES**	___ ___ ___	___ ___ ___	___ ___ ___	___ ___ ___	___ ___ ___	___ ___ ___	
COOL DOWN ACTIVITY							
# OF MINUTES TO GET HR DOWN TO 100	___	___	___	___	___	___	
STRETCHING #SECONDS HELD EACH STRETCH	___ ___	___ ___	___ ___	___ ___	___ ___	___ ___	
TOTAL MINUTES							
THOUGHTS (ABOUT YOUR WO) - BEFORE							
- DURING							
- AFTER							

CLIENT _____ Exercise Classification _____ Consultant _____

AEROBIC EXERCISE LOG   Week # _____   Intensity _____ - _____ Duration _____ - _____ Frequency _____ - _____

DAY/DATE								
WARM UP ACTIVITY								
MINUTES	‖	‖	‖	‖	‖	‖	‖	
HR								
WORK OUT ACTIVITY								
HR@1/2 WAY	‖	‖	‖	‖	‖	‖	‖	
HR@ END	‖	‖	‖	‖	‖	‖	‖	
TOTAL MINUTES								
COOL DOWN ACTIVITY								
# OF MINUTES TO GET HR DOWN TO 100	‖	‖	‖	‖	‖	‖	‖	
STRETCHING #SECONDS HELD EACH STRETCH	‖	‖	‖	‖	‖	‖	‖	
TOTAL MINUTES								
THOUGHTS (ABOUT YOUR WO) - BEFORE								
- DURING								
- AFTER								

CLIENT _____ Exercise Classification _____ Consultant _____

AEROBIC EXERCISE LOG   Week # _____   Intensity _____ - _____   Duration _____ - _____   Frequency _____ - _____

DAY/DATE						
WARM UP ACTIVITY						
MINUTES						
HR						
WORK OUT ACTIVITY						
HR@1/2 WAY						
HR@ END						
TOTAL MINUTES						
COOL DOWN ACTIVITY						
# OF MINUTES TO GET HR DOWN TO 100						
STRETCHING #SECONDS HELD EACH STRETCH						
TOTAL MINUTES						
THOUGHTS (ABOUT YOUR WO) - BEFORE						
- DURING						
- AFTER						

18

Resting Heart Rate

Your Resting Heart Rate (RHR) is a good indicator of your cardiorespiratory fitness. To take your RHR, use the radial (wrist) or carotid (neck) artery and count your pulse for a **FULL 60 SECONDS**, starting with ZERO. Do not use your thumb to take your pulse because it also has a pulse and will result in an inaccurate reading. **Take your RHR twice every day and average the two together.** At the end of the week average the 7 RHRs. The best time to take a RHR is in the morning before you get out of bed. If you are unable to get a reading in the morning, you can take a reading in the evening when you have been inactive for 30 minutes or longer (ex. After studying, reading, or lying down).

Week #5	Mon	Tue	Wed	Thurs	Fri	Sat	Sun	Average
RHR								
AM/PM								
Time of Day								
Place								

Week #6	Mon	Tue	Wed	Thurs	Fri	Sat	Sun	Average
RHR								
AM/PM								
Time of Day								
Place								

Week #7	Mon	Tue	Wed	Thurs	Fri	Sat	Sun	Average
RHR								
AM/PM								
Time of Day								
Place								

Week #8	Mon	Tue	Wed	Thurs	Fri	Sat	Sun	Average
RHR								
AM/PM								
Time of Day								
Place								

RHR _____

EHR @ 50% ___|___ @ 60% ___|___ @ 70% ___|___ @ 75% ___|___ @ 80% ___|___ @ 85% ___|___.

GOALS:

		Aerobic				Resistance Training			
Week	Activity	Intensity	Duration	Frequency	Type	Frequency	#Exercises	Sets	Reps
5									
6									
7									
8									

Summary:

RHR _____

AEROBIC EXERCISE LOG

CLIENT _____   Exercise Classification _____   Consultant _____

Week # _____   Intensity _____ - _____   Duration _____ - _____   Frequency _____ - _____

DAY/DATE						
WARM UP ACTIVITY						
MINUTES RPE/HR						
WORK OUT ACTIVITY						
RPE/HR@1/2 WAY RPE/HR@ END **TOTAL MINUTES**						
COOL DOWN ACTIVITY						
# OF MINUTES TO GET HR DOWN TO 100						
STRETCHING #SECONDS HELD EACH STRETCH						
TOTAL MINUTES						
THOUGHTS [ABOUT YOUR WO]						

AEROBIC EXERCISE LOG   Week # _____   Intensity _____ - _____   Duration _____ - _____   Frequency _____ - _____

DAY/DATE						
WARM UP ACTIVITY						
MINUTES RPE/HR	___ / ___	___ / ___	___ / ___	___ / ___	___ / ___	___ / ___
WORK OUT ACTIVITY						
RPE/HR@1/2 WAY RPE/HR@END **TOTAL MINUTES**	___ / ___ / ___ / ___	___ / ___ / ___ / ___	___ / ___ / ___ / ___	___ / ___ / ___ / ___	___ / ___ / ___ / ___	___ / ___ / ___ / ___
COOL DOWN ACTIVITY						
# OF MINUTES TO GET HR DOWN TO 100	___	___	___	___	___	___
STRETCHING #SECONDS HELD EACH STRETCH	___ ___	___ ___	___ ___	___ ___	___ ___	___ ___
TOTAL MINUTES						
THOUGHTS (ABOUT YOUR WO)						

CLIENT _____ Exercise Classification _____ Consultant _____

AEROBIC EXERCISE LOG   Week # _____   Intensity _____ - _____ Duration _____ - _____ Frequency _____ - _____

DAY/DATE								
WARM UP ACTIVITY								
MINUTES RPE/HR	__/__	__/__	__/__	__/__	__/__	__/__	__/__	__/__
WORK OUT ACTIVITY								
RPE/HR@1/2 WAY RPE/HR@ END **TOTAL MINUTES**	__/__ __/__ __	__/__ __/__ __	__/__ __/__ __	__/__ __/__ __	__/__ __/__ __	__/__ __/__ __	__/__ __/__ __	__/__ __/__ __
COOL DOWN ACTIVITY								
# OF MINUTES TO GET HR DOWN TO 100	__	__	__	__	__	__	__	__
STRETCHING #SECONDS HELD EACH STRETCH	__ __	__ __	__ __	__ __	__ __	__ __	__ __	__ __
TOTAL MINUTES								
THOUGHTS (ABOUT YOUR WO)								

25

AEROBIC EXERCISE LOG   Week # _____   Intensity ____ - _____   Duration ____ - _____   Frequency ____ - _____

DAY/DATE							
WARM UP ACTIVITY							
MINUTES RPE/HR	___/___	___/___	___/___	___/___	___/___	___/___	___/___
WORK OUT ACTIVITY							
RPE/HR@1/2 WAY RPE/HR@ END	___/___ ___/___	___/___ ___/___	___/___ ___/___	___/___ ___/___	___/___ ___/___	___/___ ___/___	___/___ ___/___
TOTAL MINUTES	___	___	___	___	___	___	___
COOL DOWN ACTIVITY							
# OF MINUTES TO GET HR DOWN TO 100	___	___	___	___	___	___	___
STRETCHING #SECONDS HELD EACH STRETCH	___	___	___	___	___	___	___
TOTAL MINUTES	___	___	___	___	___	___	___
THOUGHTS (ABOUT YOUR WO)							

RHR _____

EHR @ 50% ___ | ___ @ 60% ___ | ___ @ 70% ___ | ___ @ 75% ___ | ___ @ 80% ___ | ___ @ 85% ___ | ___ .

GOALS:

	Aerobic				Resistance Training				
Week	Activity	Intensity	Duration	Frequency	Type	Frequency	#Exercises	Sets	Reps
9									
10									
11									
12									

Summary:

RHR _____

Client _____

Month _____ Yr _____

Month _____ Yr _____

Client _____

Month _____ Yr _____

☐	☐	☐	☐
☐	☐	☐	☐
☐	☐	☐	☐
☐	☐	☐	☐
☐	☐	☐	☐
☐	☐	☐	☐
☐	☐	☐	☐

Client _____

Month _____ Yr _____

RESISTANCE TRAINING LOG

Muscle Group	Lift	Day/Date									
		Set(s)	Reps	Weight	Set(s)	Reps	Weight	Set(s)	Reps	Weight	
Legs	Press										
	Extension										
	Curls										
	Abd/Add										
Calves	Raises										
Back	Pull Down										
	Row										
	Extension										
Triceps	Kickbacks										
	Extension										
	Dips										
Chest	Bench Press										
	Chest Press										
	Incline										
	Fly										
	Cables										
Biceps	Curls										
	Hammers										
	Machine										
Shoulders	Shrugs										
	Press										
	Raises										
Abdominal	Crunches										
	Raises										

RESISTANCE TRAINING LOG

Muscle Group	Day/Date Lift	Set(s)	Reps	Weight	Set(s)	Reps	Weight	Set(s)	Reps	Weight	Set(s)	Reps	Weight
Legs	Press												
	Extension												
	Curls												
	Abd/Add												
Calves	Raises												
Back	Pull Down												
	Row												
	Extension												
Triceps	Kickbacks												
	Extension												
	Dips												
Chest	Bench Press												
	Chest Press												
	Incline												
	Fly												
	Cables												
Biceps	Curls												
	Hammers												
	Machine												
Shoulders	Shrugs												
	Press												
	Raises												
Abdominal	Crunches												
	Raises												

RESISTANCE TRAINING LOG

Muscle Group	Day/Date Lift	Set(s)	Reps	Weight	Set(s)	Reps	Weight	Set(s)	Reps	Weight	Set(s)	Reps	Weight
Legs	Press												
	Extension												
	Curls												
	Abd/Add												
Calves	Raises												
Back	Pull Down												
	Row												
	Extension												
Triceps	Kickbacks												
	Extension												
	Dips												
Chest	Bench Press												
	Chest Press												
	Incline												
	Fly												
	Cables												
Biceps	Curls												
	Hammers												
	Machine												
Shoulders	Shrugs												
	Press												
	Raises												
Abdominal	Crunches												
	Raises												

RESISTANCE TRAINING LOG

Muscle Group	Day/Date Lift	Set(s)	Reps	Weight	Set(s)	Reps	Weight	Set(s)	Reps	Weight	Set(s)	Reps	Weight
Legs	Press												
	Extension												
	Curls												
	Abd/Add												
Calves	Raises												
Back	Pull Down												
	Row												
	Extension												
Triceps	Kickbacks												
	Extension												
	Dips												
Chest	Bench Press												
	Chest Press												
	Incline												
	Fly												
	Cables												
Biceps	Curls												
	Hammers												
	Machine												
Shoulders	Shrugs												
	Press												
	Raises												
Abdominal	Crunches												
	Raises												

RESISTANCE TRAINING LOG

Muscle Group	Lift	Day/Date													
		Set(s)	Reps	Weight	Set(s)	Reps	Weight	Set(s)	Reps	Weight	Set(s)	Reps	Weight	Set(s)	Reps
Legs	Press														
	Extension														
	Curls														
	Abd/Add														
Calves	Raises														
Back	Pull Down														
	Row														
	Extension														
Triceps	Kickbacks														
	Extension														
	Dips														
Chest	Bench Press														
	Chest Press														
	Incline														
	Fly														
	Cables														
Biceps	Curls														
	Hammers														
	Machine														
Shoulders	Shrugs														
	Press														
	Raises														
Abdominal	Crunches														
	Raises														

RESISTANCE TRAINING LOG

Muscle Group	Day/Date Lift	Set(s)	Reps	Weight	Set(s)	Reps	Weight	Set(s)	Reps	Weight	Set(s)	Reps	Weight
Legs	Press												
	Extension												
	Curls												
	Abd/Add												
Calves	Raises												
Back	Pull Down												
	Row												
	Extension												
Triceps	Kickbacks												
	Extension												
	Dips												
Chest	Bench Press												
	Chest Press												
	Incline												
	Fly												
	Cables												
Biceps	Curls												
	Hammers												
	Machine												
Shoulders	Shrugs												
	Press												
	Raises												
Abdominal	Crunches												
	Raises												

EVALUATION OF AEROBIC EXERCISE PROGRAM

Student _____ Consultant _____

<u>Circle the appropriate evaluation for each:</u>

Compliance   Met the ACSM guidelines listed below:
Aerobic 3-5 X week/ 30-60 minutes/ 50-85%
Resistance Training 2-4 X week/ (full body)

                  A - 8 weeks or longer
                  B - 7 weeks
                  C - 6 weeks
                  D - 5 weeks
                  F - 4 weeks or less
                             50% _____

Records (logs)   A - 12 weeks
                  B - 11 weeks
                  C - 10 weeks
                  D - 9 weeks
                  F -   8 weeks or less
                             25% _____

Pre/Post Tests   A - Completed
                  C - Completed one
                  F - Did none
                             25% _____

_____

Date _____ **EXERCISE PROGRAM GRADE** _____
_____

Attitude toward aerobic exercise?

Benefits for including aerobic exercise in your schedule:

Program you will follow now that your class is over:

Confidence in maintaining this program (10 - very high; 1 - none)   _____

GUIDELINES FOR SELF HEALTH BEHAVIOR MODIFICATION

1. Pinpoint (select an <u>EXACT</u> behavior - is it measurable?]

2. Log current behavior for baseline information before we start to change [How many? How much? Situations? Anecdotes]

3. Select a meaningful reward [Is it feasible? Is it powerful? Can it be given immediately to a successful behavior, or systematically in a plan?]

   Schedule of Reinforcement ["Schedule" the changes, "Reinforce" each success]:

4. Start small [The first step must be a bite that can be chewed.]

5. Gradually increase the desired behavior and/or decrease the reward.

   Environmental or external factors contributing to success:

   Avoid situations typically preceding negative behavior.

   Enlist support of friends or family, find substitute behaviors

43

SELECTING A HEALTH SELF-BEHAVIOR
MODIFICATION PROJECT

Assessment	OK	Needs Improvement	Major Change Required
1. Food group deficiencies?			
2. Fiber deficiency?			
3. Blood chemistry indications?			
a. Total cholesterol			
b. LDL-cholesterol			
c. HDL-cholesterol			
d. Triglycerides			
e. Glucose			
4. Stress assessment?			
5. High blood pressure?			
6. Pre-lifestyle assessment?			
a. Stress			
b. Alcohol			
c. Fitness			
d. Nutrition			
e. Tobacco			
f. Safety			

7. Does your Family History task from the course manual give you any ideas for possible project topics? List possible behaviors.

8. Does the textbook Figure 10.4, Self-Assessment of risk factors for coronary heart disease, give you any ideas for possible project topics? List possible behaviors.

IS CHANGING A HEALTH BEHAVIOR EASY?

PICK A TOUGH ONE AND THINK ABOUT IT!

1. Below, write two health behaviors you think you should change. Don't pick easy ones, but instead choose behaviors which your study tells you would enhance your long-term health and well-being.

2. Ask your neighbor if you have stated your health behaviors in such a way that s/he could tell you how it could be measured. From your discussion, write how you could measure each of the health behaviors you've chosen. **Be specific.**

3. Now, fill out at least five items on the page titled "These Are a Few of My Favorite Things," and fill in the blanks beside each one. Below, write down 2 possible rewards that would help you change one of the above health patterns.

Next, determine if the behaviors you've chosen should be changed suddenly and all at once (cold turkey smoking cessation, for example), or, as Mark Twain said, "Habit is habit, and not to be thrown out the window all at once, but coaxed downstairs one step at a time." If your behaviors should be changed gradually, and many should, then write down a number of steps which would change your behaviors gradually.

THESE ARE A FEW OF MY FAVORITE THINGS

This exercise will help you to select meaningful rewards to aid you in your health behavior change program.

STEP 1.   On the chart below, list 10 things you like best to do.

THINGS I LIKE TO DO BEST	$	P	X	F	Po	AF
				1	1	1
				2	2	2
				3	3	3
				4	4	4
				5	5	5
				6	6	6
				7	7	7
				8	8	8
				9	9	9
				10	10	10

STEP 2.   For the first three columns after your list, do the following:

a. In the first column, write a $ sign next to the things costing more than $3 every time you do them.

b. In the second column, write "P" next to the things you must do with other people.

c. In the third column, write "X" next to the things that you feel are important for the person you like best.

STEP 3.   In the last three columns, circle the numbers for items which meet the following criteria:

a. [F] FEASIBLE. It would be possible for me to do this or use this as a reward.

b. [Po] POWERFUL. I would work for this reward. It would be a good incentive.

c. [AF] ADMINISTER FREQUENTLY. I could earn this reward or accumulate parts of this reward, frequently, or soon after a successful step on my B-mod plan.

BEHAVIOR MODIFICATION PROJECT LOG

Client _____ Consultant _____

Current Behavior _____ Goal Behavior _____

Date _____   1.   Summary of discussion:

                                  Goals for next week:

Date _____   2.   Summary of discussion:

                                  Goals for next week:

Date _____   3.   Summary of discussion:

                                  Goals for next week:

Date _____   4.   Summary of discussion:

                                  Goals for next week:

Date _____   5.   Summary of discussion:

                                  Goals for next week:

Date _____   6.   Summary of discussion:

                                  Goals for next week:

Date _____   7.   Summary of discussion:

                                  Goals for next week:

Date _____   8.   Summary of Project:

EVALUATION OF BEHAVIOR MODIFICATION PROJECT

Student _____ Consultant _____

Circle the appropriate evaluation for each:

Progress

A - Met goals every week
B - Met goals (6 out of 8 weeks)
C - Met goals (5 out of 8 weeks)
D - Met goals (4 out of 8 weeks)
F - Met goals fewer than 4 weeks

50% _____

Records (logs)

A - 8 weeks - creative and very detailed - typed
B - 7 weeks - Good detail - typed
C - 6 weeks - hand written, minimum information
D - 5 weeks - hand written information
F - 4 weeks or less - information recorded less
than minimum requested

25% _____

Reward system

A - Very effective/creative
C - Acceptable
F - Not used

25% _____

Date _____ **BEHAVIOR MODIFICATION PROJECT GRADE** _____

What progress did you make?

What benefits did you receive from making this change?

What is your confidence level in maintaining your new habit: (10 - very high; 1 - none)? _____

HEALTHY LIFESTYLES
STUDY GUIDE: TO YOUR HEART'S CONTENT

1. What is <u>a</u>erobic exercise?

   cardiovascular exercise, steady, rythmic, continuous

2. How do you calculate your maximum heart rate? What is yours?

   220 - Age ; 199

3. According to Dr. William Haskell of the Stanford Heart Disease Prevention Program, what is the talk test?

   conversation, during exercise good

4. To take your exercise heart rate, you should count your pulse for how long?

   10 sec × 6

5. Dr. Haskell states that a beginning exerciser could alternate vigorous (target zone) activity with easier exercise until the target zone is sustainable for 10 minutes. Then he suggests that a person could increase target zone activity per session by how many minutes per week? Until how many minutes are achieved?

   1 min ; at least 20 mum

6. The moderate view suggests that a person with multiple risk factors for heart disease should do what before beginning an exercise program?

   See a doctor

7. Stretching helps to avoid what?

   ↑ flexibility. change btwn nod. +

AEROBICS & ANAEROBICS

Aerobic exercise is exercise in which oxygen is used during the

muscular contractions - the aerobic pathway.

> Vacation - Go now, pay now

What are some examples of aerobic exercise?

Anaerobic exercise is exercise in which oxygen is not used during the

muscular contractions - the anaerobic pathway.

> Vacation - Go now, pay later

What are some examples of anaerobic exercise?

MAXIMUM OXYGEN CONSUMPTION

The maximum volume of oxygen that a person can burn per kilogram of

body weight per minute (Max VO_2/KG/min) is the best indicator of

cardiovascular fitness. This is sometimes expressed as "METS."

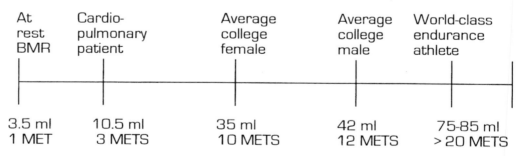

At rest BMR	Cardio-pulmonary patient	Average college female	Average college male	World-class endurance athlete
3.5 ml 1 MET	10.5 ml 3 METS	35 ml 10 METS	42 ml 12 METS	75-85 ml > 20 METS

At rest (BMR) we burn 3.5 ml/KG/min, and the average college female (at exhaustion) is capable of energy expenditures 10 times resting, the average college male 12 times resting, and top endurance athletes 20 to 25 times resting oxygen consumption rates.

HHP 100: HEALTHY LIFESTYLES

Interview an exerciser.   Name _____

What is your future image?   Due Date _____

Part I: (Turn in Parts I and II on a separate piece of paper.)

Talk with a person you consider to be an exercise "nut." In general, try to determine what
they do, why they do it, what motivates them, etc. Some potential areas for questions you
might ask them are listed below. If you can think of additional questions - go right ahead
and ask. Jot down their responses or a summary of your conversation with them. We will
discuss these in class.

   1.   What type of exercise do they do?

   2.   Why did they get started?

   3.   Why did they stay with it? What benefits do they receive?

   4.   What is the hardest part?

   5.   Has exercise become a part of them? If so, in what ways?

Part II:

In the U.S.A. today, the average person will live into their 70's, and some will live into their
80's and beyond. To begin our thinking about aging and the accompanying quality of life,
project your self ahead 30 years.

Where do you believe your current lifestyle health behaviors will lead you in 30 years?
What will you look like? What will you expect of yourself in terms of physical activity?
What will your overall health and quality of life be like? Can you think of any changes you
could make now which would enhance this image you have of yourself in 30 years?

HEALTH TIP: Warming Up

by Dr. John Scheer, Associate Professor

Years ago I could walk onto a racquetball court, a tennis court, or the first tee and fire away without even taking a warmup swing. For jogging I was warmed up in half a lap. I can't do that anymore. Now the sole purpose of the first mile of a jog is to get rid of the creaks and the rust, and is it ever slow! If I teed off without a warmup, my body feels like it would shatter into a thousand pieces and crumble to the ground like you'd imagine a glass breaking from a high pitched sound. My friends (?) smilingly tell me it's just the aging process and that it happens to everybody as they reach middle age. To me, it's simply a reminder of the importance of a warmup.

You can design a warmup to fit your needs. It should take you from an inactive state to your most vigorous intensity gradually and slowly. If you are going to play racquetball, arrive 10 minutes early to stretch out before your court time starts. Slow, static stretching is better than bouncing, which only triggers a reflex which is counter productive to getting the muscle stretched out. When you take the court, warm up easily at first, gradually increasing the intensity until you're ready to play.

Stretching is also an important part of a cool down. For prevention of chronic low back problems, pay particular attention to stretching the hamstrings and the muscles of the low back. After a cool down stretching session, situps may help with low back health also. Keep your knees bent and do slow curls with no head or arm whip to give you momentum. It is not important to go all the way up, but it is important that the abdominal muscles initiate the curl.

How will you benefit from a proper warmup and cool down? First, you may prevent an acute injury to the muscles or joints from starting too fast. Second, you probably will help prevent chronic low back pain, which can be a debilitating thing.

There may be yet a third benefit, which could become critical as we get a little older. The importance of a warmup was described by Dr. William Haskell, Co-Director of the Stanford University Heart Disease Prevention Program and Cardiac Rehabilitation Program, who visited the UN-L campus as a keynote speaker for our first annual Wellness Week. A cardiac rehab program at a major California hospital was experiencing one cardiac event (heart attack) for each 5,000 hours of patient exercise, while the national average was one per 30,000 hours of exercise. Haskell served on a team which examined the program. The only way this hospital differed from established practice was that they allowed patients to come in an time during the stretching and warmup time instead of demanding prompt arrival for the entire warmup. When the patients were required to be on time for the warmup in order to participate, the program went right to the national average for heart attacks during rehabilitation.

One intervention note: when Dr. Haskell was here, we went for a 4 mile jog. We went to the locker room, changed, went out to the track, and I said "Are you ready?" He said, "You bet!", and immediately began stretching for 10 minutes! So do yourself a favor. Give yourself a little extra time for warming up and cooling down. The benefits are worth it.

HEALTH TIP: WATER LOSS

Dr. John Scheer

Water is an extremely important, but often forgotten, nutrient for athletes and exercisers. According to Dr. Ann Grandjean, Chief Nutritional Consultant for the US Olympic Committee, a loss of just 2-3% of body weight during activity can reduce oxygen utilization, aerobic power, speed, coordination, and judgment. A cumulative water loss of 3-4% over several days will result in the same performance decrements.

Evaporation of sweat is your body's main method of cooling itself. Failure to replace lost water slows your sweating, and therefore the cooling of your body. Exercise in high humidity slows the evaporation of sweat, resulting in the same reduction in cooling efficiency.

So, if you want to perform your best in athletics, exercise, or sports participation, the following suggestions may help.

1. Weigh yourself before and after exercise to determine how much water you should drink to replace lost fluid. A two pound weight loss would require four 8-ounce glasses of water. Weighing will also enable those people who are heavy sweaters, and therefore at greatest risk for poor performance as well as heat illness, to identify themselves.

2. After you have determined what your water needs are, you should drink before, during, and after exercise or competition. Drink water as close to the beginning of a workout as possible. For extended activity, 3-5 ounces of cold water each 10-15 minutes during workouts is recommended.

3. In hot weather, wear one layer of light, loose, absorbent clothing. Throw away your rubberized workout gear, and use your other sweatsuits only in colder weather. I was jogging on a hot, humid morning recently and observed another jogger run for 40 minutes in black sweatpants and black sweatshirt with the hood up and tied. The man may not have been a fool, but he certainly was ignorant.

4. Do not take extra salt. We get more than enough sodium in our normal diet. Excess sodium simply pulls water out of cells resulting in dehydration and, in some people, increased interstitial fluid, blood volume, and blood pressure.

5. Water is emptied from the stomach and absorbed through the small intestine rapidly, which is what we want. Sports drinks that contain small concentrations of electrolytes (e.g. 100 mg. of sodium in 20 ounces) and carbohydrates are also good. Do not use alcohol, caffeinated drinks, or pop for water replacement.

In addition to these suggestions, the elderly and children need to take special care to drink adequate water. The thermoregulatory system does not work as well in the elderly. Children have a greater surface area per body mass, less sweat overall and per sweat gland, and take longer to acclimate. For each 40 kilograms (88 pounds) of body weight, children should drink 5 ounces of cold water each 30 minutes.

Finally, thirst is not your best indicator of your need for water. the body will undergo what is called voluntary dehydration. That is, by the time you are thirsty, you will already be somewhat dehydrated, and performance may be affected. The recommendation that is made to Olympic athletes, and it applies to all of us, is "never become thirsty."

How much weight will you lose during your next workout?

HEALTH TIP: EXERCISE ADDICTION
Dr. John Scheer

In America we seem to have the mind set that if something is good for you, more of it must be better. Exercise is often viewed this way. We have discussed the health benefits of exercise, and, for those so inclined, an abundance of articles are available which extol the virtues of a highly active lifestyle.

Some readings, however, remind us that more is not necessarily better where exercise is concerned. Richard Greene, in "Does Physically Fit Mean Fiscally Fit?" in Forbes Magazine (9/22/1986), discussed corporate executives who exercise. Even though some research has shown a positive relationship between fitness and academic performance, Greene cited examples of fit executives with poor job performance, and called attention to muscular and skeletal injuries which can result from overexercising. Physical fitness does not automatically lead to superior work, and chronic medical problems are a potential outcome of overdoing it. Even Dr. Kenneth Cooper, popularly called the "Father of Aerobics," has stated that anybody who jogs more than about 15 miles per week is doing so for some reason other than health benefit.

In The Body of America, Blair Sabol attacks the notion of exercising for hours each day to achieve some elusive goal called physical perfection. She believes that many people enter an exercise program without clear cut goals, then become addicted and consumed by their program. Contrary to popular belief (or hope), we cannot eliminate the inevitable aging process through an enormously time-consuming fitness addiction. She further believes that some people who become addicted to exercise are using it as an escape - from relationships, for example. She writes, "I was so exhilarated by my new sense of physical strength that my friends and lovers became secondary considerations in my life and eventually vanished from it. I was independently bionic, so who needed people?"

If your goal for participating in an exercise program is primarily to maintain health and vigor, and reduce your risks of cardiovascular disease, then this is just a reminder. If you exercise 4 to 5 times a week for 30 minutes or so per session, at 70 to 85% of Maximum heart rate, you are achieving most of the health benefits available through aerobic exercise. The intensity should be moderate, certainly not exhaustive. Include some slow, static stretching activities to maintain low back health and some recreational strength conditioning to build and maintain muscle mass, and you've got a good program. Good luck!

STRENGTH

AN IMPORTANT COMPONENT OF PHYSICAL FITNESS
FOR OLD AND YOUNG ALIKE!

Dr. John Scheer and Professor Jan Callahan

When it comes to our lean muscle mass, the research overwhelmingly supports the old axiom "use it or lose it!" Each of us should develop a modest, or recreational, strength conditioning program as part of a truly healthy living pattern.

We start to lose lean muscle mass and strength in our mid 20s, especially inactive people. Problem is, we probably don't take notice until we're a little older and find ourselves unable to do things we used to just take for granted. The vicious cycle of a gradual decrease in activity levels breeding a loss of muscle mass, which leads to further inactivity and further muscle loss leads to such popular bumper stickers as "When you get older, sit happens!" It also leads to one of the most common reasons for older folks having to go to nursing homes because they no longer have enough muscle strength to take care of themselves, as happens when one loses the ability to get up out of a chair (or toilet seat) without help. In this condition, quality of life can go in the toilet, so to speak.

Lean muscle mass really drives metabolic rate. Muscle tissue burns 10 times as many calories as fat tissue. Thus, the number of calories we burn while at rest is based on how much muscle mass we have. Further, creeping obesity is exaggerated by a loss of muscle which results in a decrease in resting metabolic rate.

This diminished quality of life does not have to happen, or at the very least it can be delayed until quite an old age and mitigated in the meantime. What is required is a lifetime commitment to a modest strength program, one that can be accomplished with a relatively small weekly time commitment if designed properly. Following are a few ideas to supplement the textbook material we've already read.

1. **FREQUENCY**. 2 - 3 sessions per week on non-consecutive days.

2. **MODE**. Select 8-10 resistance training machines distributed across lower body, upper body, and middle body muscle groups. Vary the exercises occasionally. Big muscle groups should always be a focus of your program (ie back, chest, leg muscles, etc)!

3. **INTENSITY.**
    a. Do 10-12 repetitions per set to muscle fatigue. Trial and error can determine how much weight results in muscle fatigue after 10-12 reps.
    b. Do 1-3 sets per muscle group with 1 or 2 minutes rest between sets. Two or 3 sets is good, but even 1 set provides significant change.

4. **CAUTION**. Beginners should start small. To avoid excessive soreness, do not go to muscle fatigue the first several weeks. By then trial and error determination of weight will be easier.

5. **BENEFITS.**
    a. Build lean muscle mass when young. Look good. A good start on lifetime weight control.
    b. Maintain muscle mass or slow the rate of loss in the middle years. Help avoid "creeping obesity."
    c. Maintain adequate strength for high quality of life in older years. Maintain independence or reduce dependence on others. Maintain active lifestyles for both enhanced quality of life and for reduction of chronic disease risk.

LDL - CHOLESTEROL

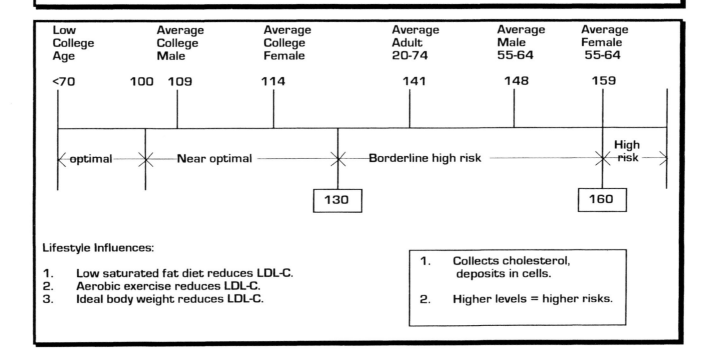

Lifestyle Influences:

1. Low saturated fat diet reduces LDL-C.
2. Aerobic exercise reduces LDL-C.
3. Ideal body weight reduces LDL-C.

1. Collects cholesterol, deposits in cells.
2. Higher levels = higher risks.

TOTAL CHOLESTEROL

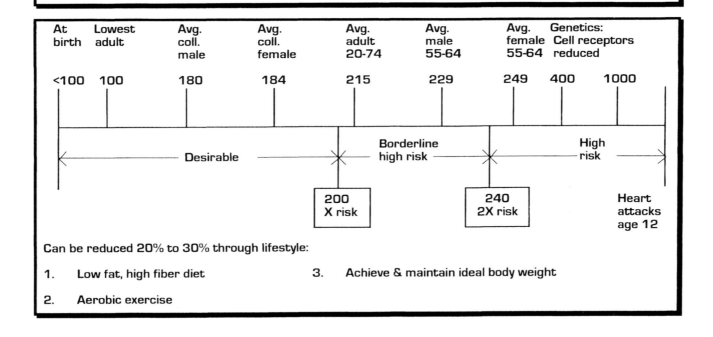

Can be reduced 20% to 30% through lifestyle:

1. Low fat, high fiber diet
2. Aerobic exercise
3. Achieve & maintain ideal body weight

HDL - CHOLESTEROL

Steroid use?	High risk	Average male	Average female	Low risk	Long-lived?
15-25	<40	45	53	≥60	75+

Facts about HDL-cholesterol:

1. The higher the better, protects us from CHD, higher levels = lower risk
2. Picks up cholesterol, transports it from sites of excess for removal.

Lifestyle influences:

1. Aerobic exercise increases HDL-C.
2. Smoking reduces HDL-C.
3. Steroid use can reduce HDL-C.

HDL - RATIO

1. The HDL-ratio is a calculation indicating the proportion of our total cholesterol that is bound to high-density proteins (HDL).

2. Divide your total cholesterol by your HDL-cholesterol.

3. The lower this number, the better (the more HDL you have).

4. What is the HDL-ratio in each example below, and which is better?

   a. T.C. = 200, HDL-C = 33   b. T.C. = 200, HDL-C = 66

5. Men should be below 4.5, women below 4.0.

6. Ideal is below 3.5.

7. Lifestyle influences include aerobic exercise, low fat diet, weight control, smoking.

FOLLOWING UP A CHOLESTEROL TEST

A. CLASSIFICATION*

1. < 200 mg/dl   Desirable Blood Cholesterol
2. 200-239 mg/dl   Borderline-High Blood Cholesterol
3. ≥240 mg/dl   High Blood Cholesterol

B. RECOMMENDED FOLLOW-UP

1. Total Cholesterol <200 mg/dl ──────────→ Repeat within 5 years

2. Total Cholesterol 200-239 mg/dl

    a. **Without definite CHD or two or more other CHD risk factors (See "Count Your Risks")──→ Dietary information and recheck annually

    b. ***With definite CHD or two or more other CHD risk factors (one of which can be male sex)──────────────→

3. ****Total Cholesterol ≥ 240 mg/dl ────→

2b. or 3:
See physician;
Lipoprotein analysis;
further action based on
LDL-cholesterol level

*   The directors of the National Cholesterol Education Program have stated that all adults should try to achieve a serum cholesterol level of less than 200 mg per deciliter of blood. Levels between 200 and 239 mg are associated with an increased risk of cardiovascular disease, while levels above 240 are termed "high risk".

**   If you are in category 2a above, you are encouraged to implement dietary suggestions and re-check your cholesterol in one year (and perhaps have your HDL and LDL fractions tested).

***   If you are in category 2b above, you are encouraged to see your physician to verify the results and have your HDL and LDL cholesterol fractions tested.

**** If you are in category 3 above, you are strongly encouraged to see your physician to verify the results and have your HDL and LDL cholesterol fractions tested.

CHD Risk Factors: Male sex, family history, smoking, hypertension, low HDL-C < 40 mg, diabetes, cerebrovascular or occlusive peripheral vascular disease, severe obesity > 30% overweight.

COUNT YOUR RISKS

To determine the initiation level for treatment, people in the borderline high risk group (total cholesterol 200-239 mg/dl; LDL-C 130-159 mg/dl) need to count their additional risk factors. Two or more of the following indicates the need for lipoprotein analysis and physician visit:

1. Am I a male?

2. Do I have a parent, brother or sister who has suffered a heart attack or sudden death before age 55?

3. Do I smoke cigarettes?

4. Do I have high blood pressure?

5. Is my HDL-Cholesterol below 35 mg/dl?

6. Do I have diabetes mellitus?

7. do I have definite cerebrovascular or peripheral vascular disease?

8. Am I severely obese (30% or more overweight)?

TRIGLYCERIDES

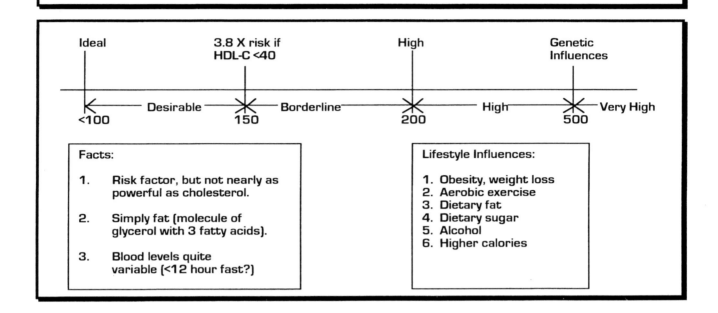

Ideal	3.8 X risk if HDL-C <40	High	Genetic Influences

←———— Desirable ————X———— Borderline ————X———— High ————X———— Very High

<100   150   200   500

Facts:

1. Risk factor, but not nearly as powerful as cholesterol.

2. Simply fat (molecule of glycerol with 3 fatty acids).

3. Blood levels quite variable (<12 hour fast?)

Lifestyle Influences:

1. Obesity, weight loss
2. Aerobic exercise
3. Dietary fat
4. Dietary sugar
5. Alcohol
6. Higher calories

GLUCOSE

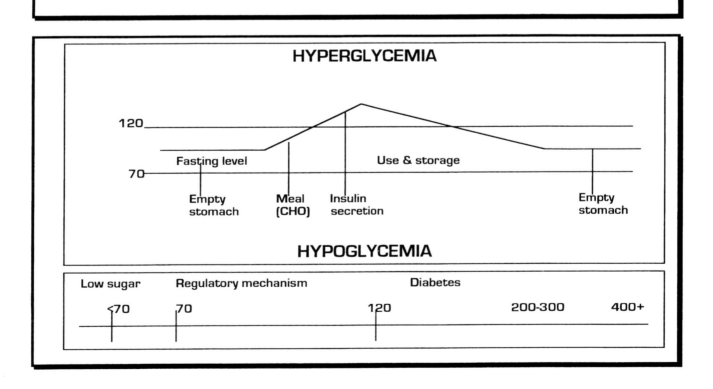

HYPERGLYCEMIA

120 ——————————————————————

Fasting level   Use & storage

70 ——————————————————————

Empty stomach   Meal (CHO)   Insulin secretion   Empty stomach

HYPOGLYCEMIA

Low sugar	Regulatory mechanism	Diabetes		
<70	70	120	200-300	400+

NUTRITION RULE #1:

EAT A BALANCED DIET

WHICH INCLUDES A VARIETY OF FOODS

SUGGESTED SERVINGS		SIZE OF SERVINGS
MILK GROUP		1 minimum serving =
Children	3 servings per day	8 ounces (1 cup) - milk, buttermilk or skim milk, yogurt
Teens	4 servings per day	1 1/3 ounce - cheese
		1/2 cup - cottage cheese
Adults	3 servings per day	1/2 cup - ice cream
MEAT GROUP		1 minimum serving =
2 servings per day		3 ounces - meat, cooked (not including bones or fat)
increase size or number of servings for teen-agers, mothers-to-be and nursing mothers		2 ounces - luncheon meats 2 tablespoons - peanut butter 2 eggs 1 cup - dried peas or beans, cooked
FRUITS		1 minimum serving =
*2-4 servings per day		1/2 cup cooked 1/2 cup juice
1 source of Vitamin C every day 1 source of Vitamin A 3 to 4 times per week		1 medium-sized orange 1/2 medium grapefruit, or 1/4 cantaloupe
VEGETABLES		1 minimum serving =
*3-5 servings per day		1/2 cup cooked 1/2 cup juice 1 medium sized potato
BREADS AND CEREALS		1 minimum serving =
*6-11 servings per day		1 slice bread 1 ounce ready-to-eat cereal 1/2 cup cooked cereal, corn meal, grits, macaroni, spaghetti, rice

*For 2,000 calorie diets, a minimum of 2 fruits, 3 vegetables, and 6 breads and cereals is recommended. For 2,500 calorie diets the middle range is recommended, and for 3,000+ calorie diets the upper end of the ranges is recommended.

24 HOUR RECALL

On the form below, follow the directions presented in class. If known, beside food items record <u>specific</u> brand names; fast foods; cereals; preparation (fried, baked, broiled, boiled); added mayo, lettuce, tomato, sauces, dressings, cheeses, margarine, etc.; and other characteristics, such as "reduced fat", "reduced salt", etc.

	Food Items	# Servings of each	Total # of Servings	Grams of Dietary fiber
FRUITS specify juice or whole fruit	1. peach 2. 2 slices cantaloupe 3. juice 4. 5. 6.	4/3 2-4	Fruit servings = _____ _____ _____	Fruit fiber = 9 _____ _____
VEGETABLES Include beans, peas, nuts	1. potato, 2. broccoli 3. broccoli 4. carrots 5. 6. 7.	4 3-5	Vegetable servings = _____ _____	Vegetable fiber = 12 _____ _____
GRAIN PRODUCTS Specify whole grain or white flour products	1. bagel 2 serving 2. cashew cheese 3. mixed nuts 4. oatmeal 5. granola bar 6. 7. 8. 9. 10. 11.	6 11	Grain servings = 8 _____ _____	6 Grain fiber 8 3 = _____ 8
MILK Specify % fat	1. soy milk 2. 3. 4.		Milk servings = _____	
MEAT Fowl: specify with or without skin	1. 2. 3.		Meat servings = _____ _____	

How should we record calorie containing items that do not fit into the 5 food groups?

F _____
A _____
S   cookie _____

My total dietary fiber in the last 24 hours was _____ grams.
The USA average is _____ grams.
The American Cancer Society recommends _____ grams.

NUTRITION RULE #2: EAT A SMART FAT DIET

A HOW ARE CALORIES FIGURED?

1   Trim N' Lite yogurt contains 10 grams of protein, 17 grams of carbohydrate, and 2 grams of fat in a one cup, 8 ounce, serving. How many calories, then are in one serving? _____

What three "givens" must you know to answer this question?

a. _____

b. _____

c. _____

2   One serving, or 3 ounces, of T-bone steak contains 20 grams of protein and 20 grams of fat. A 12-ounce T-bone, therefore, has how many calories? _____ What percent of its total calories are fat? _____

3   If you would like further practice on problems such as these, select any food item from Appendix B at the back of the text, note the grams of protein, CHO, and fat per serving and calculate the total calories _____, and the % fat _____.

B FOCUS ON FAT

1   The average American consumes 37% fat. If the average college female consumes around 2000 calories per day, and the average male around 2500 calories, how many grams of fat per day does the average college female eat? _____ The average college male? _____

2   We should eat less than 30% fat. Keeping the calories constant, how many grams of fat should we cut from the diet to go from 37% to 29%?

Females? _____   Males? _____

3   Again, using the charts at the back of the text, if a person had two servings of whole milk in a day, and he or she were to switch to skim milk, how many grams of fat would he or she cut from the daily intake? _____

2% to skim? _____   2% to 1%? _____

4   We could solve similar problems focusing on saturated fat. Why are palm and coconut oils, sometimes called the tropical oils, considered bad?

5   If a person wanted to gain weight, what should he/she do in regard to:

a   Exercise _____?

b   Protein intake _____?

c   Fat intake _____?

66

REDUCE DIETARY FAT?

In class, we calculated that a 20 gram per day reduction in dietary fat would take most of us from the U.S.A. average of 37% fat to the recommended 30% or less. How hard would this be to achieve?

With 3 required servings from the milk group, what kind do you drink? How much could you reduce dietary fat just through this food group?

Macronutrient	Whole Milk	2% Milk	1% Milk	Skim Milk
Protein	8 G	8 G	8 G	8 G
Carbohydrate	11 G	11 G	11 G	11 G
Fat	8 G	5 G	3 G	1 G

What is <u>your</u> potential fat reduction just from milk?

What about other milk products (cottage cheese, ice cream, cheese)?

FISH: IS IT REALLY THAT GOOD?

YES! EVEN HIGH FAT FISH!

Dr. John Scheer

Have you read lately about the health benefits of eating fish? Nutritionists have been recommending fish as a good, healthy food for a long time. Most fish is lower in fat, which means that protein supplies a greater proportion of the calories, than red meat. And, after all, we eat the meat group primarily for protein, not fat.

Studies have shown that the health benefits of fish may be even greater than previously thought. It has been found that large populations of people who consume a lot of fish have significantly less cardiovascular disease than people who do not eat much fish. The fat in fish oil is largely polyunsaturated, which is better than the saturated fat in red meat. Perhaps more important, however, are the presence of Omega-3 fatty acids, a special kind of polyunsaturated fatty acid, found in fish. The Omega-3 fatty acids reduce the stickiness of blood platelets, reducing both the clotting ability of blood and the gradual buildup of arterial plaque, thus reducing obstruction of arteries and the formation of clots which can be life threatening. Thus, high fat fish is enjoying a good reputation now. So eat some salmon, mackerel and herring!

Those populations noted above with low levels of heart disease risk consume large quantities of fish. If you are interested in a dietary change which may reduce your heart disease risk, both the Harvard Medical school Newsletter and the University of California, Berkeley Wellness Letter recommend consuming at least two to three servings of fish per week.

Find some fish recipes that you like, then make them part of your regular diet. It may take some experimenting, but in the long run it would be well worth it. Here's a recipe you might like. Buy or catch some white fish, then simmer it in lemon juice until it turns white and flaky. Put the fish in a shallow casserole dish, add some chopped onion, a little margarine, and some seasoning on top, then broil it until it turns brown and crispy on top. It's delicious and even kids like it!

Be careful with fast food fish and fish sandwiches. Some of them contain more added fat than hamburgers have! Also, health food zealots have jumped into the marketplace with fish oil supplements and pills. The current state of research knowledge is not adequate to support the use of these supplements, and consumers should not be taken in by advertising claims. For now, reduce stress in your life by taking a kid fishing, then eat what you catch! Good luck!

HEART DISEASE RISK FACTORS

Of the 2.2 million people who die each year in the USA, cardiovascular (cardio = heart; vascular = blood vessels) diseases still claim the most victims, many of them prematurely, for both women and men.

Lifestyle plays a major role in the development of heart disease, and much can be done to prevent it, slow it down, or delay its onset.

Below, write down the risk factors which predispose people to the development of heart disease. Identify which ones are primary, and how much each one increases risk. Also, which ones are either partially or totally within our control? Which ones are beyond our control?

Risk Factors/Predisposing Influences (Primary? Secondary? Controllable? Uncontrollable?)

WOMEN & HEART DISEASE

By age 55, women are as likely as men to develop high blood pressure. By 65, women have a higher risk than men.

Men remain more likely than women overall to have heart attacks, but women have a much higher rate of strokes.

A woman age 55 who smokes and has high blood pressure and elevated cholesterol has a one-third higher risk of heart attack than a man age 55 with the same 3 risk factors.

More than half of all women over 55 have blood cholesterol levels above 240, the level at which CHD is high risk.

Cigarette smoking poses a greater risk for women. A woman age 55 who smokes is in more danger of heart attack than a man age 55 who smokes.

American Heart Association

NUTRITION RULE #3:

EAT A DIET THAT IS LOW IN SUGAR

Dr. John Scheer

Table sugar or sucrose, is a simple carbohydrate (CHO) which is devoid of nutrients beyond the calories per gram, or empty calories, it contains. Excessive sugar can play a role in diabetes, obesity, heart disease, and malnutrition, to name just a few.

In the first decade of the 21st century, we find the USA lifestyle has now lead to (1) dramatic increases in childhood obesity, (2) alarming increases in the diagnosis of ADULT onset diabetes in CHILDREN, and (3) epidemic overweight and obesity in adults. Might this be a reason that some school districts and States are considering laws and policies to eliminate pop machines from schools? Vending machines dispensing pop at 9 teaspoons of sugar per can, are NOT in the best interests of kids!

Complete these calculations for class:

1. The average American consumes 125 pounds of sugar per year. If one pound contains 454 grams, how many sugar calories per day does the average American eat? _____

2. If we average around 2400 calories per day, what % of our total calories is sugar? _____

3. What is the average % fat in the USA diet? _____

4. Add together the average % fat and average % sugar. Of all the calories consumed in the USA, today, fat and sugar account for what percent? _____

5. We often eat sugar in processed foods that we don't even know is there. Dr. Sharon Balters, a former nutritionist in the Center for Healthy Lifestyles, said that if you find a product that lists sugar as one of the first three ingredients of the label, it probably has a fair amount of sugar and you can probably do better, or find a better product in the same food group with less sugar. Examine some labels for sugar (sucrose) content. What kinds of products do you typically eat that have a lot of sucrose? What alternatives might be better?

NUTRITION RULE #4: EAT A DIET HIGH IN FIBER
ESTIMATING DIETARY FIBER INTAKE

Dr. John Scheer

Fiber is the indigestible parts of plant products (carbohydrates) we eat. It is abundant in whole fruits, vegetables, and whole grain products. It is less abundant in fruit juices and white flour products because some of the fiber has been removed in processing.

The average American eats 12 grams of fiber per day, which contributes to a host of chronic diseases (from cancer to heart disease, hemorrhoids to diverticulitis and varicose veins) which are prevalent in developed countries today. Soluble fiber slows glucose absorption and binds cholesterol in the intestine, helping reduce blood cholesterol and manage diabetes. Insoluble fiber binds water, making fecal content softer and bulkier so it can pass through intestines more quickly and easily. The American Cancer Society and dietetic associations recommend 25 to 35 grams per day.

Fiber is included in food labels, and labels can be used when available. But we can also estimate fiber intake as long as a person eats a variety of foods from day to day:

FRUITS	**3 grams** of fiber per whole fruit	Fruits average almost 3 g if we don't count cantaloupe and watermelon, which have almost no fiber. They vary, so eat a variety!
VEGETABLES	**3 grams** per serving	Again, this is average and they vary, so eat a variety.
WHOLE GRAIN BREADS	**1.5 grams** per serving	Bread, pasta, brown rice, etc.
WHOLE GRAIN CEREALS	**4 grams** per serving	They vary quite a bit, so labels can help
WHITE BREAD	**1/2 gram** per serving	Bread, pasta, white rice
WHITE FLOUR CEREALS	**0 to 1 gram** per serving	Fiber is mostly gone

What is a serving?   Fruits   1 piece of fruit, 1/2 grapefruit, handful of grapes

Vegetables: 1/2 cup or 1 big serving spoon full

Breads: 1 slice, 1/2 cup pasta or rice or 1 big serving spoon

Cereals: 1 ounce, or a normal breakfast bowl of cereal

DIETARY SODIUM IS EVERYWHERE!

IS TOO MUCH BAD FOR YOU?

Sodium is an electrolyte which helps maintain water balance in the body. We only need a few hundred milligrams a day, but the average American consumes more than 5,000 milligrams (5 grams), most of it in the form of salt. Salt is 40% sodium and 60% chloride.

Dr. Jean Mayer, former nutritionist at Harvard, stated, "There is not the slightest doubt in my mind that high sodium intake predisposes to hypertension" (high blood pressure). The human species evolved as a sodium conserving organism, as salt was a rare commodity. We have forced our bodies, through high intakes, to be sodium sloughers, however. About 20% of us, it is estimated, do not do well in sloughing excess sodium, and our blood pressure increases with high sodium intake. More recent evidence indicates that we may become increasingly sensitive to sodium as we reach our 40s and 50s, and blood pressure increases with age are common in our country.

High blood pressure (140/90, either number being higher on repeated measurements) is associated with increased risk of stroke, heart disease, congestive heart failure, kidney problems, and eye problems. Part of the problem is that hypertension has no symptoms (it has been called the silent killer), and many people, when diagnosed, must be on blood pressure medication the rest of their lives.

The government nutrition guidelines recommend that adult Americans limit sodium intake to 2400 milligrams per day. Remember, we add about 1/3 of all the sodium we eat at the table and in cooking, about 1/6 occurs naturally in the foods we eat, and fully 1/2 is in processed food we buy. We can reduce or eliminate optional salt in recipes, and comparing food labels can be a huge help.

It is helpful to develop a sense for sodium quantities which are low, moderate, and high, and reading food labels can help with this also. The food charts at the back of the textbook, Appendix B, list sodium for a wide variety of foods from each food group. Using Appendix B in the textbook and your 24 hour recall assessment we completed in class, how many milligrams of sodium did you have?

HYPERTENSION

HYPERTENSION IS SOMETIMES CALLED THE SILENT KILLER.

IT INCREASES THE RISK OF:

1. STROKE

2. HEART ATTACK

3. EYE DAMAGE

4. KIDNEY FAILURE

5. HEART FAILURE

ESSENTIAL HYPERTENSION

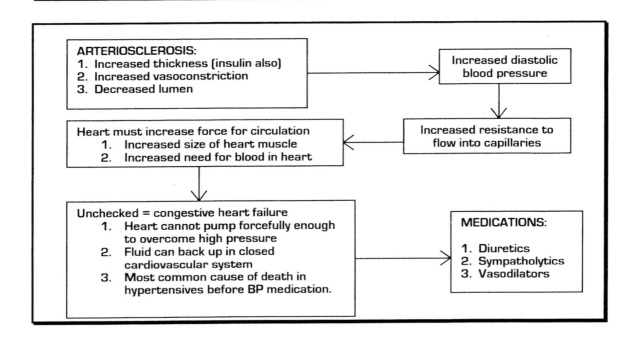

ARTERIOSCLEROSIS:
1. Increased thickness (insulin also)
2. Increased vasoconstriction
3. Decreased lumen

Increased diastolic blood pressure

Heart must increase force for circulation
1. Increased size of heart muscle
2. Increased need for blood in heart

Increased resistance to flow into capillaries

Unchecked = congestive heart failure
1. Heart cannot pump forcefully enough to overcome high pressure
2. Fluid can back up in closed cardiovascular system
3. Most common cause of death in hypertensives before BP medication.

MEDICATIONS:

1. Diuretics
2. Sympatholytics
3. Vasodilators

EFFECTS OF SALT

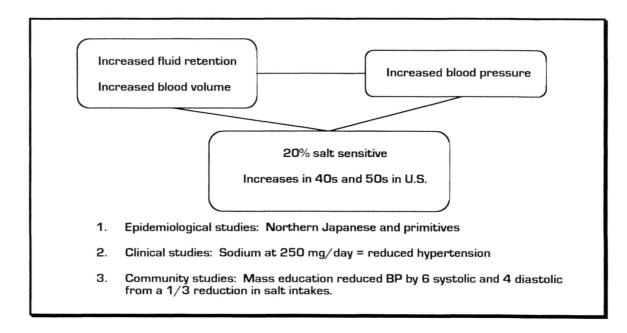

Increased fluid retention

Increased blood volume

Increased blood pressure

20% salt sensitive

Increases in 40s and 50s in U.S.

1. Epidemiological studies: Northern Japanese and primitives

2. Clinical studies: Sodium at 250 mg/day = reduced hypertension

3. Community studies: Mass education reduced BP by 6 systolic and 4 diastolic from a 1/3 reduction in salt intakes.

SODIUM

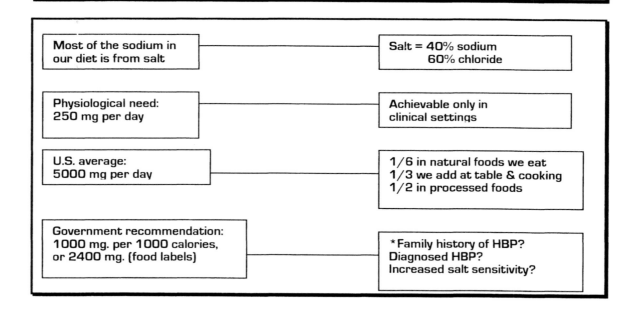

Most of the sodium in our diet is from salt

Salt = 40% sodium
          60% chloride

Physiological need:
250 mg per day

Achievable only in
clinical settings

U.S. average:
5000 mg per day

1/6 in natural foods we eat
1/3 we add at table & cooking
1/2 in processed foods

Government recommendation:
1000 mg. per 1000 calories,
or 2400 mg. (food labels)

*Family history of HBP?
Diagnosed HBP?
Increased salt sensitivity?

SODIUM IN LOW-PROCESSED FOODS

Food group	Minimum Servings	Avg. Sodium per serving	Total Sodium
Meat	_____	_____	_____
Milk	_____	_____	_____
Grains	_____	_____	_____
Fruits	_____	_____	_____
Vegetables			
Totals			_____

If we eat good foods from the 5 food groups, sodium is at the low end.

Where does our 5,000 mg average intake of sodium come from?

Consult your textbook charts and food labels.

HIGH BLOOD PRESSURE:

WHAT CAN I DO?

High blood pressure, sometimes called the silent killer, is a significant problem in this country, affecting close to 60 million Americans. High blood pressure can affect the brain, heart, and kidneys, and even mild high blood pressure can speed up arteriosclerosis and other problems which lead to chronic disease.

What can be done? First, a person should have his or her blood pressure monitored regularly. As with most chronic disease problems, early detection can be helpful. Second, many research studies have shown the following lifestyle related habits to be effective in reducing high blood pressure in some people.

1. Get regular aerobic exercise.

2. Reduce salt intake.

3. Achieve ideal weight.

4. Regularly practice a formal relaxation technique.

5. Don't smoke.

6. If medication is prescribed, by all means take it as directed.

LIFETIME WEIGHT CONTROL

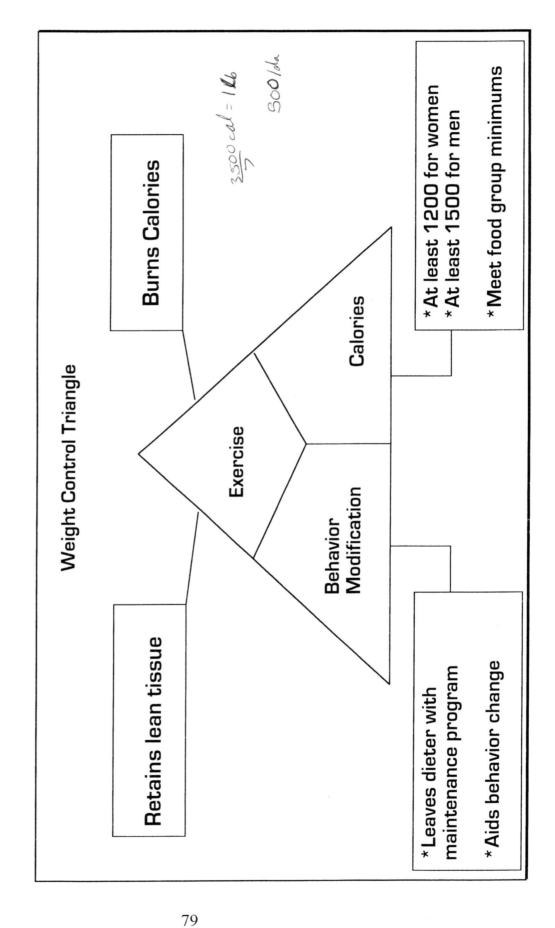

Weight Control Triangle

Burns Calories

Retains lean tissue

Exercise

Behavior
Modification

Calories

$\dfrac{3500 \text{ cal} = 1 \text{lb}}{7}$

500/da

* Leaves dieter with
  maintenance program

* Aids behavior change

* At least 1200 for women
* At least 1500 for men

* Meet food group minimums

140

THE MATHEMATICS OF WEIGHT CONTROL
Healthy Lifestyles, Dr. John Scheer

You will need to answer several types of questions involving the arithmetic of weight control on both a quiz and the final exam for Healthy Lifestyles. Bring a calculator!

A.   First, nutritionists and exercise physiologists make the obvious observation that exercise burns calories, and can, therefore, contribute to a calorie deficit that will cause the body to lose weight. A rough, ballpark figure is that we burn about 100 calories per mile on foot. Since 3500 calories = 1 pound, it takes around 35 miles of jogging or walking to burn 1 pound. If a person jogged or walked 12 miles a week for a year, how many pounds worth of calories would that person burn?

        1.   100 (calories/mile) X 12 (miles/week) = 1200 (calories/week)
        2.   1200 (calories/week) X 52 (weeks/year) = 62400 (calories/year)
        3.   62400 (calories/year) ÷ 3500 (calories/pound) = 17.83
(pounds/year)

B.   If a person jogged or walked 2 miles a day, and reduced calorie intake by 425 calories per day, how much weight should that person lose in one week?

        1.   2 (miles/day) X 100 (calories/mile) = 200 (calories/day)
        2.   425 (calories/day) + 200 (calories/day jog/walk) = 625 (calorie
deficit/day)
        3.   625 (calorie deficit/day) X 7 (days/week) = 4375 (calorie deficit/week)
        4.   4375 (calorie deficit/week) ÷ 3500 (calories/pound) = 1.25
(pounds/week)

C.   A young man weighed 200 pounds and was found, through body composition assessment, to be 25% fat. He wanted to be 18% fat, because his health professor said that would be healthier. What should he weigh? The formula to follow is:

$$\frac{LBW\ (Lean\,Body\,Weight)}{1.0 - Desired\%\,fat}$$

In the above formula, desired % fat should be expressed as a decimal (e.g. 18% = .18). The steps to follow to solve the problem are:

        1.   200 (pounds) X .25 (% fat) = 50 (pounds of fat)
        2.   200 (pounds) - 50 (pounds of fat) = 150 (pounds of lean, or LBW above)
        3.   150 (LBW) ÷ 1.00 - .18 (desired % fat) = 150/.82 = 183 (pounds)

D.   A young lady weighs 140 pounds and is 30% fat. She begins a moderate, recreational strength conditioning program. After 6 months, she weighs 136 pounds and is 25% fat. How did her lean weight change? How did her fat weight change? With simple subtraction, you can calculate these changes after just doing the following:

        1.   140 (pre-pounds) X .30 (pre % fat) = 42 (pre pounds of fat)
        2.   136 (post-pounds) X .25 (post % fat) = 34 (post pounds of fat)

FAD DIETS

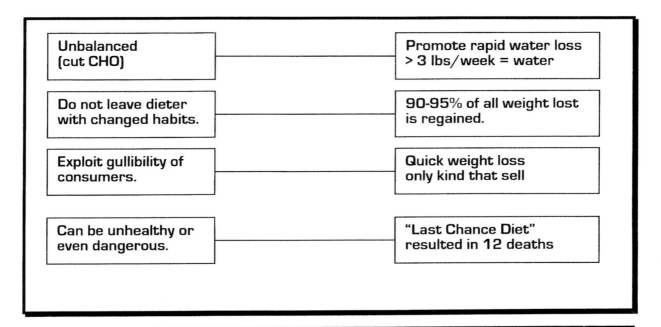

Unbalanced (cut CHO)	Promote rapid water loss > 3 lbs/week = water
Do not leave dieter with changed habits.	90-95% of all weight lost is regained.
Exploit gullibility of consumers.	Quick weight loss only kind that sell
Can be unhealthy or even dangerous.	"Last Chance Diet" resulted in 12 deaths

HEALTHY WEIGHT LOSS

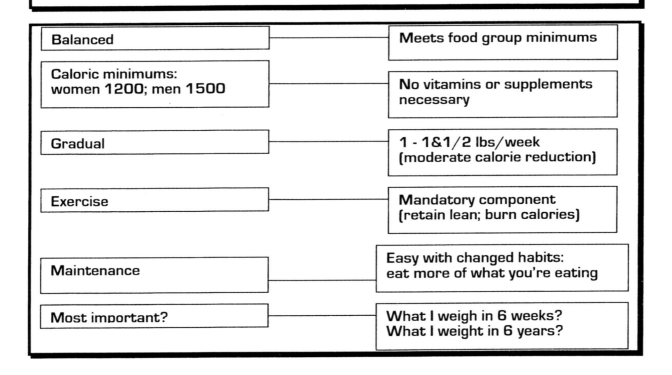

Balanced	Meets food group minimums
Caloric minimums: women 1200; men 1500	No vitamins or supplements necessary
Gradual	1 - 1&1/2 lbs/week (moderate calorie reduction)
Exercise	Mandatory component (retain lean; burn calories)
Maintenance	Easy with changed habits: eat more of what you're eating
Most important?	What I weigh in 6 weeks? What I weight in 6 years?

REDUCING RISK
Reducing the risk for alcohol-related problems *

Each year, millions of Americans experience negative consequences as a result of drinking alcohol. In fact, just about all of us have at one time or another experienced an alcohol-related problem, or know someone who has. Some of the more common negative consequences related to drinking "too much" include personal health problems, drunk driving arrests and crashes, family problems, inability to perform at work, and endangering your safety as well as the safety of others.

In light of the many serious problems that alcohol abuse can cause, many people are making the decision to "drink responsibly." But what exactly do phrases such as "drink in moderation," "drink responsibly," or "know when to say when" actually mean? Dr. Ernest Noble, Director of the UCLA Alcohol Research Center, states that, "these are emotionally appealing but ambiguous phrases. They can mean anything one wants them to mean - from almost total abstinence to not falling over the cat when tiptoeing in from a late drinking bout."

So, is there really such a thing as responsible drinking? This is a difficult question to answer. Given the fact that alcohol has known anesthetic, cell-damaging, and psychoactive properties (not to mention having addictive capability), it is important to understand that drinking is far from a risk-free activity. Thus, the question becomes: "How can we reduce the risk of experiencing an alcohol-related problem?"

The answer is as easy as 0-1-2-4!

"by the Numbers: 0-1-2-4" is an easy to understand alcohol use formula. If followed consistently, the "By The Numbers" formula helps individuals greatly reduce their risk for experiencing an alcohol-related problem.

Let's take a closer look at the formula, number by number.

0 The first number in the formula is "zero." "Zero" represents the recommendation of no alcohol use, or abstinence. Research, circumstantial evidence, and common sense suggest that there are certain situations where any alcohol use may increase the risk for negative outcomes, and there are some groups of people for whom drinking may represent significant risk.

These recommended times to abstain can be easily remembered by the acronym OBSERVE, which stands for:

> **O**n certain medications or have certain illnesses.
> **B**ehind the wheel or engaged in tasks that require full mental or physical functioning.
> **S**tressed or tired.
> **E**ither the son, daughter, or sibling of someone with alcoholism.
> **R**ecovering from alcoholism or drug dependence.
> **V**iolating existing laws, policies, or personal values.
> **E**xpecting, nursing, or considering pregnancy.

In order to reduce the risk of experiencing an alcohol-related problem, it is important to appropriately follow the "zero" category guidelines. For some people, the recommendation of "zero" will apply for a lifetime (for example, people with a family history of alcoholism), while for others the recommendations will apply only periodically (for example, women who are pregnant or those who are under the legal drinking age).

The rest of the "By The Numbers" formula applies to those who do not fall into the "zero" category and choose to drink. It is important to understand that the "By The Numbers" formula is designed to help those who choose to drink decrease their risk for experiencing either short-term and/or long-term alcohol-related problems. This does not imply that those who presently abstain need to start drinking in order to comply with the formula. For those who do not presently drink, there is no research suggesting that they should start now.

*By Dr. David Hunnicutt, Robert C. Schroeder, & Maggie Mann, Alcoholism and Drug Abuse Council of Nebraska. Reproduced with permission.

1 "One" stands for no more than one standard drink per hour. A "standard" drink is defined as one that contains one-half ounce of pure alcohol. This is the approximate amount one would find in a 12-ounce beer, a four-ounce glass of table wine, or a one-ounce shot of 100-proof distilled spirits. This is important information because the "average" individual will metabolize approximately one-half ounce of alcohol per hour–the equivalent of one "standard" drink.

If an individual consumes more than one "standard" drink per hour, or consumes drinks that are higher in alcohol content than those previously mentioned, the risk for experiencing an alcohol-related consequence is increased because alcohol is being consumed at a rate faster than the body can metabolize it. As a result, while the excess alcohol waits for its turn to be metabolized, it keeps circulating in the bloodstream and produces impairment and possibly even physical damage.

2 The "two" in the formula stands for no more than two drinks per day for men, one for women. These are the amounts which, if exceeded, are associated with long-term health problems such as cardiovascular disease, certain cancers, liver disease, pancreatic disease, neurological and psychiatric disorders, and a host of other diseases, including alcoholism.

Research is indicating strongly that women experience problems after consuming less alcohol than men over shorter periods of time. For this reason, the recommendation is lower for women than for men (more on that in a minute).

4 The "four" in the formula stands for no more than four days per week. Many times, when people consume alcohol, it initially gives them feelings of pleasure. As a result, some people tend to increase their use of alcohol, striving to gain that positive feeling they associate with using alcohol. Unfortunately, if this happens frequently over a period of time, a dependent relationship with alcohol can begin to develop. In order to reduce the risk of this type of relationship developing, it is recommended that individuals interject regular periods of abstinence by consuming alcohol no more than four times per week.

CAVEATS

Again, it is important to understand that the "By The Numbers" formula is designed to help those who choose to drink decrease their risk for experiencing either short-term and/or long-term alcohol-related problems. This does not imply that those who presently abstain need to start drinking in order to comply with the formula. For those who do not presently drink, there is no research suggesting that they should start now.

Further, these alcohol use recommendations are hourly, daily, and weekly limits. For this reason, there is no option to "save up" drinks. Saving up "allowed" drinks and consuming them all in one evening would undoubtedly increase an individual's likelihood of experiencing an alcohol-related consequence and, therefore, is not an option in the formula.

"A STANDARD DRINK"

Not all drinks are created equal. The alcohol found in beer, wine, and distilled spirits is ethanol. A standard drink contains one-half ounce of ethanol–the amount you would find in a 12-ounce beer, a one-ounce shot of 100-proof distilled spirits, or a four-ounce glass of table wine. Generally, this is the amount of ethanol which an individual can metabolize in about an hour.

This is important information because some drinks may have more than one-half ounce of alcohol. This means that some drinks are equivalent to more than one drink. For example, some wine coolers have nearly twice the alcohol content as a "standard" drink.

Also, it is important to remember that experts recommend sipping drinks as opposed to gulping them or "slamming" them.

ALCOHOL AND WOMEN: CRITICAL INFORMATION

Current research indicates that women are not as efficient "drinking machines" as males. In other words, men and women do not respond to alcohol in the same way. There are a variety of factors which influence this difference.

The first factor is body size. Equivalent doses of alcohol produce higher levels of concentration in smaller individuals. On the average, women are of smaller build than men.

The second factor is body composition. It appears that the average female carries more body fat than the average male, and body fat contains little water. Alcohol, when consumed, dilutes uniformly into body water. Thus, given the same body size, the average female has less body water to dilute the alcohol. This produces a higher concentration for a female than for a male, even if both drink the same amount and are the same size.

The third factor is a metabolizing enzyme called alcohol dehydrogenase. This enzyme helps the body to rid alcohol from the system. Women have less of this enzyme than men do. Thus, more of what they drink enters the bloodstream in the form of pure alcohol.

Finally, preliminary research suggests that the menstrual cycle and use of oral contraceptives (because of the change in hormones) may intensify a woman's response to alcohol.

Because of these differences, women can expect substantially more impairment than men at equivalent doses. In addition, preliminary research findings suggest that alcohol problems among women may develop as a result of shorter drinking histories than men, and may be more severe.

For these reasons, to reduce the risk for experiencing alcohol-related problems, it is recommended that women limit their consumption to no more than one drink per hour, no more than one drink per day, and no more than four times per week.

Remember, this is a **HEALTH** issue, not an equality issue.

SUMMARY

The information in these guidelines, if consistently followed, should help individuals greatly reduce their risk for experiencing short-term impairment problems, long-term health-related problems, or both.

It is important to understand that if an individual sincerely tries to follow the "By The Numbers" guidelines, but finds that he or she cannot consistently do so, it is recommended that an alcohol counselor be contacted. Although it does not necessarily mean that a problem is present, the matter does warrant further attention.

Alcohol: Attitudes, but Consequences

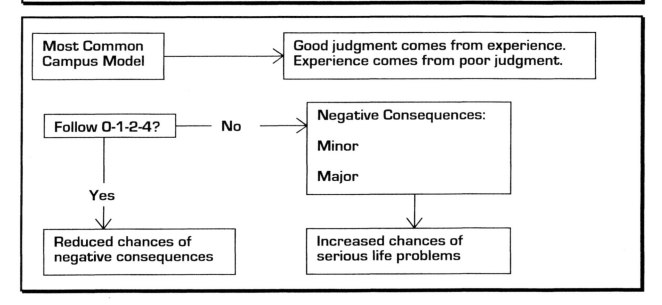

Most Common Campus Model → Good judgment comes from experience. Experience comes from poor judgment.

Follow 0-1-2-4? — No → **Negative Consequences:** Minor / Major

Yes ↓

Reduced chances of negative consequences

Increased chances of serious life problems

FRIGHTENING FACTS

1. On Friday and Saturday nights, one out of every 10 cars coming toward you has a drunk driver behind the wheel.

2. On other nights of the week, one out of every 50 drivers is drunk.

3. Teenage drivers cause five times as many highway deaths in the United States as drivers in the 35 - 64 age group.

4. Male teenagers have the worst driving record of any group in the nation.

5. Of the 25,000 alcohol-related deaths on American highways last year, 35% of the victims were in the 16 - 24 age group.

IS IT WORTH THE RISK?

SEXUALLY TRANSMITTED DISEASES

STUDY GUIDE NOTES & QUOTES

A   STDs: What are the odds?
1   Sexually transmitted diseases are the third most common infection in the United States after colds and flu. STDs are especially common among people under the age of 25.
2   The Centers for Disease Control has declared sexually transmitted diseases as epidemic for people aged 15 to 29 years of age.
3   The STD epidemic is nothing new. Did you know that during the Civil War it is thought that more soldiers suffered from STDs than were wounded or killed? In World War II more soldiers were treated for STDs than were treated for battle injuries.
4   We know that people who are at risk for becoming infected with a sexually transmitted disease, such as chlamydia or genital warts, are also at risk for getting HIV.
5   the risk for HIV infection is greater in those who have been infected with other STDs because many of the risk behaviors are similar and some STDs create lesions or sores in tissues of the vagina or penis through which the HIV can enter.
6   An estimated 15 million people get an STD EACH YEAR.
7   2/3 of those who get an STD are under age 25.
8   What do these two facts really mean for the college age population?
   a   Multiply 15 million times a 4.5 year college career.
   b   Multiply the result times .67.
   c   What are the odds of STD infection on a college campus?

B   What kinds of STDs might risk behaviors lead to?
1   STDs that are caused by <u>bacterial infection</u> are treatable and curable with the use of antibiotics.
   a   Some infections respond differently to certain antibiotics. An antibiotic that you are given to treat your bronchitis won't necessarily be effective for an STD.
   b   It is important that you never attempt to self-medicate or treat yourself if you think you may have an STD. Always seek medical care.
   c   Bacterial infections can be prevented by the use of latex condoms.

2   <u>Parasitic infections</u> can also be treated and cured.
   a   While scabies and pubic lice are difficult to prevent spreading if one partner is infected with them, trichomoniasis can be prevented through the use of condoms because the protozoa live inside the vagina and/or the urethra.
   b   it is very important that both partners are treated when an STD is diagnosed. Just because one partner doesn't have symptoms doesn't mean they are not infected.
   c   If both partners are not treated then the Ping-Pong effect can occur where partners just keep passing the infection back and forth to each other.

3   STDs caused by <u>viruses</u> cannot be cured. Once you are infected, you are infected for life.
   a   Between as many as 20-40 million Americans are infected with genital warts. Genital warts can be removed, but because the virus is always in the body, they can grow back and the HPV virus can be transmitted to partners.
   b   At least 31 million Americans are infected with genital herpes. Most symptoms of herpes outbreaks can be relieved with medication, however, for some sufferers the effects can be quite painful.

c   Additionally, HPV and Herpes are related to a higher risk for cervical cancer in women and create risk to newborns during childbirth. Very often mothers who have genital warts or herpes deliver their babies by C-section.

d   Hepatitis B causes damage to the liver which can lead to chronic liver disease and death. 1.5 million people carry Hepatitis B.

e   HIV is the virus that causes AIDS. It is estimated that over 1 million Americans are infected with HIV. We can't know for sure because being HIV positive is not a reportable disease to the centers for Disease Control. Only the diagnosis of AIDS is a reportable condition.

C   What are some common sexually transmitted diseases?
1   Bacterial - Can be cured
   a   Chlamydia
   b   Gonorrhea
   c   Syphilis
   d   Chancroid

2   Parasites - Can be removed
   a   Pubic Lice
   b   Scabies
   c   Trichomoniasis

3   Viral - 4 H's - No Cure: These will be your friends for LIFE!
   a   HPV - Genital Warts
   b   HSV 1 & HSV 2 - Herpes
   c   HBV - Hepatitis B
   d   HIV - Human Immuno-deficiency Virus

D   What are some of the symptoms? What should I look for?
1   Any of the symptoms should be examined by a health care professional. It is always better to have something checked out - better safe than sorry.

2   Remember just because the symptoms go away doesn't mean you are free from infection. Some STD symptoms disappear only to reoccur later with more serious consequences.

3   People with active cases of STDs (for example, chlamydia, gonorrhea, herpes or syphilis) are three to five times more likely to get HIV because these infections damage the membranes of the reproductive system which can allow HIV to enter the body.

4   STD symptoms
   a   Unusual discharge from penis or vagina
   b   Burning or pain during urination
   c   Discomfort during intercourse
   d   Unexplained bleeding
   e   Bumps, blisters, pimples, sores, lesions, rash, odor, itching, or swelling

5   Any of these symptoms should be examined by a physician.

E   Are there gender differences?

1   In general men are more likely to...
   a   notice symptoms because their reproductive organs are on the outside of the body.
   b   think they are not at risk for STDs.

    c   infect a partner.

2 Women and STDs
    a   A woman is twice as likely as a man to contract an STD from one act of unprotected sex with an infected partner.
    b   Up to 75% of women experience no symptoms of an STD infection compared to 25% of men.
    c   About 150,000 women each year become infertile as a result of pelvic inflammatory disease (PID). PID is a complication of STDs that go untreated or where treatment is delayed.
    d   Cervical cancer is more associated with genital herpes and genital warts.
    e   In general, women are more easily infected, less likely to have symptoms, and more likely to have frequent and severe health problems.
    f   Infertility is just a word, but what would it really mean to someone?

F HIV in the USA: The CDC has given a new name to the 15 - 24 age group - "The New Susceptibles."

    1 The TRANSMISSION RATE of any virus is affected by two factors:
      a   The inherent efficiency of the virus.
      b   The encounter rate.

    2 The TRANSMISSION RATE of HIV, therefore, is affected by two conscious behaviors:
      a   Condom use = reduced virus efficiency.
      b   Abstinence or monogamy with an uninfected partner = reduced encounter rate.

    3 The experts tell us that if a person practices monogamy he or she will not get an STD. What kind of monogamy are the experts talking about?
      a   One sex partner for LIFE.
      b   <u>Serial monogamy</u> means that you remain faithful within a relationship, but may have had a few or several relationships over time.
      c   If a person has had sexual relationships with more than one partner in his or her life, he or she has an STD risk factor called multiple partners.
      d   A monogamous relationship means one sex partner FOR LIFE.
      e   If you or your current sex partner have had serial monogamous relationships - you have an STD/HIV Risk Factor called MULTIPLE PARTNERS.
      f   "Every time you sleep with someone, you are sleeping with all their partners, and all their partner's partners."
      g   The risk of acquiring HIV and STDs increases as the number of partners increases.

G ALCOHOL IS A RISK FACTOR - The research is clear:
    1 Alcohol increases the likelihood of unplanned sex.

    2 Alcohol increases the likelihood of multiple sex partners.

    3 Alcohol decreases the likelihood of condom use.

    4 Some use binges to absolve themselves of responsibility.

    5 A person would have sex with someone he/she would not even have lunch with!

H   Protecting Yourself from STDs/HIV
1   Let's be very clear about what abstinence means -
    a   It means NO FORM OF SEXUAL ACTIVITY where blood, semen, or vaginal secretions come in contact with another person. Any such activity is a risk factor.

2   ABSTINENCE IS SAFEST, of course. There are many people who delay having a sexual relationship until marriage. Some of their reasons include:
    a   Personal Values
    b   Religious teachings
    c   Emotional and Psychological Reasons
    d   Safety

3   If abstinence is not your choice then...
    a   Mutual monogamy with an uninfected partner.
    b   Communication - but remember some people may not know they are infected. And in the real world - sometimes people don't tell the truth about sexual history. Yes, some people lie to get sex.
    c   You have to ask the right questions to know if someone is at risk. It may be hard for some people to ask whether a partner has a history of IV drug use or to ask a man if he's ever had sex with another man. Another risk factor for HIV is if a person has traded sex for money or drugs. What about multiple sex partners? Unprotected sex?

4   If you are not abstinent or in a truly mutually monogamous relationship
    a   AND are sexually active ...
    b   OR plan to be sexually active ...
    c   You should use a latex condom correctly every time you have sex!!!

5   One of the greatest barriers to using condoms is what a person thinks might happen if condoms are used. Some think that:
    a   Condoms don't work - HIV can pass through them.
    b   Condoms don't feel natural.
    c   Condoms interfere with "the mood."
    d   Everything about condoms is embarrassing - buying them, talking about them, using them.
    e   Sometimes we have to separate the myth from what we expect might happen and concentrate on the benefits of protecting yourself and your partner.
    f   If you decide to be sexually active, doesn't it make sense to do so as safely as possible?

6   Condoms are Effective When Used Correctly as a Barrier to HIV!
    a   The US FDA requires that all latex condoms made in the US meet exact standards for length, width, thickness, and durability.
    b   A Latex condom must be a sufficient barrier to a water molecule. That means that a molecule of water must not be able to pass through the latex barrier.
    c   Imagine this on a mammoth scale. A sperm cell would be equivalent to the size of a train, an HIV virus would be equivalent to the size of a man, and a water molecule would be equivalent to the size of a dog.
    d   This is how latex condoms are able to be an effective barrier to the HIV virus.

7   Condom Shopping Nightmares. Is it really Mission Impossible?:
    a   It's common - you just know that you're going to run into someone you know when you need to buy some condoms.

89

b   You just want to get in and out of the store without being noticed, and wouldn't you know - you pick up a box without a price, and they call for a price check!
c   This is not the time for a pushy salesclerk, but you get one who goes through all the decisions you must make!
d   What is really likely to happen when you go into a store? Pharmacists and drug store clerks won't embarrass you.

8   When buying condoms DO
   a   There is a huge variety of latex condoms available on the market today. If you find that you don't care for one brand, try another.
   b   There is some indication that a condom made out of plastic will be on the market very soon. This is good news for people who are allergic to latex. Also, because plastic doesn't break down as easily a wider variety of lubricating products can be used.
   c   DO - buy LATEX condoms
   d   DO - buy LATEX condoms with a lubricant
   e   DO - buy LATEX condoms with a lubricant that contains nonoxynol-9
   f   DO - buy LATEX condoms with a lubricant that contains nonoxynol-9, with a reservoir tip
   g   DO - check the expiration date on the package

9   When buying condoms DON'T
   a   Remember only condoms made out of latex are effective as a barrier for HIV. Don't buy natural or lambskin sheath condoms for protection against STDs/HIV.
   b   Don't wait until you need them to buy them. Be prepared.
   c   DON'T - buy condoms made of any material other than LATEX
   d   DON'T - buy or use condoms with an expired date on the package
   e   DON'T - be shy about buying condoms - 40% are sold to women

10 Buying Condoms on Campus
   a   University Health Center Pharmacy
   b   The Residence Hall - Vending Machines. Who can tell...are you buying a Snickers or a Trojan?
       •   Abel, Cather, Harper, Schram, Smith, Selleck, Sandoz
   c   University Bookstore

CIGARETTE SMOKING:

MORE THAN JUST A HEALTH HAZARD

Healthy Lifestyles, John Scheer

LOOKING OLDER BEFORE YOUR TIME

1. Skin: For years, physicians have been saying that the skin of smokers ages faster than in nonsmokers. A study recently published now supports this claim. The skin of smokers wrinkles more than nonsmokers as they grow older, and it wrinkles sooner than in nonsmokers.

2. Hair: The hair normally grows more coarse as we age, but it grows coarser in smokers than in nonsmokers, and it grows coarser sooner as well (Dr. Garland Bare).

FOR WOMEN

1. Menopause: Smoking women enter menopause an average of four years sooner than nonsmoking women (Dr. Bare).

2. The Pill: Birth control pills and smoking can be a fatal combination. There is a huge increase in risk of heart disease for women who do both. In the 1970s this was reported to be a 55 fold increase in risk for women in their 40s (Dr. Kenneth Cooper). Today, physicians counsel women to stop smoking, and to not smoke AND take the pill in combination after age 35 (OB-Gyn. Dr. Steve Swanson and Dr. Bare).

3. Fetal HR: Fetal heart rate, normally 140 to 150 BPM, accelerates to 200-250 BPM during and after smoking. Deprived of oxygen, the heart must work harder.

4. Intrauterine Deaths: In the USA over 10,000 intrauterine deaths per year are attributed to smoking.

5. Infants: Infants born to smoking mothers (a) have lower birth weights, (b) fuss more, and (c) have a reduced appetite when compared to infants born to nonsmoking mothers. These infants are born with an addiction that cannot be satisfied, and they must suffer withdrawal from a highly addictive substance.

THE MACHO MAN?

1. Sex Drive: Although the sex drive never goes away, it does diminish somewhat as men grow older. According to Dr. Bare, the sex drive in smoking men begins to diminish 15 years sooner than in nonsmoking men! Is this the macho image promoted by the tobacco companies in their advertising?

SECONDHAND SMOKE

1. **Disease Risk:** Information is accumulating rapidly that nonsmokers who regularly breathe smoky air are at significantly increased risk of lung cancer (3,000 deaths per year in the USA), heart disease (30,000 to 50,000 deaths per year in the USA), aggravation of asthma, and impaired blood circulation.

2. Former U.S. Surgeon General Dr. C. Everett Koop was prompted to say, "It is now clear that disease risk due to inhalation of tobacco smoke is not limited to the individual who is smoking."

3. **Kids:** The children of smokers have increased risk of more colds, bronchitis and pneumonia, chronic coughs, ear infections, and reduced lung function.

4. **CO:** While carbon monoxide levels in the blood of smokers are typically 4 times normal, reducing the oxygen carrying capacity of the blood by 34%, CO levels are 2 times normal in the blood of nonsmokers exposed to secondhand smoke, and this increase in carboxyhemoglobin persists for 3 to 4 hours after leaving the smoky environment. Even in a nonsmoker exposed to secondhand smoke, the reduced oxygen carrying capacity of the blood could turn a good aerobic exercise session into a struggle.

SUMMARY

We know that smoking represents the single biggest cause of preventable death and disease in the USA today, killing some 435,000 Americans each year. From the information above, however, it is apparent that smoking is more than just a health hazard to the smoker. The tobacco industry shows us ads depicting young, beautiful people smoking and having fun. This image quickly fades, however, as smokers age more quickly than nonsmokers, develop more than 60 related diseases, and die prematurely.

Surveys of students who take Healthy Lifestyles show smoking rates of class participants to be slightly less than the national average for adult Americans. A fair number of students in any one class, however, will classify themselves as occasional smokers who only smoke in specific situations, such as a party, or with specific other people. If you fall into this category, you need to be aware of two things:

1. Nicotene is a powerfully addictive substance.

2. The literature on addiction reveals a dramatic trend from lesser amounts to greater amounts and from lesser frequency to greater frequency in the use of addictive substances.

Ask yourself this simple question: "Do I want to smoke or use tobacco the rest of my adult life?" If the answer is no, then recognize occasional smoking as an extremely risky proposition and decide to stop now, before the habit accelerates. On average, we cut smoking rates in half in this class. You know you'll never regret quitting. Good luck!

CANCER RISK REDUCTION

STUDY GUIDE

1. Which two vitamins seem to be important for cancer risk?

   A , C

2. What kinds of vegetables seem to be important for cancer risk?

   Cruceferous

3. What are some of the vegetables from #2 above?

   Cruceferous: Broccoli, cauliflower, brussels sprouts, cabbage, kale

4. What are the five protective lifestyle behaviors for cancer risk, or behaviors which should be added to the lifestyle?

   — Eat well
   — Wt. control - diet, exercise
   — no Salt cured, nitrite cured
   — No cigarette smoking
   — No alcohol

5. What are five risk factors for cancer, or behaviors which should be reduced or eliminated from the lifestyle?

   — Salt
   — cigarettes
   — alcohol
   — Sunrays

6. How many people die from cigarette smoking each year in the U.S.?

   465,000

7. What are the 7 warning signals for cancer?

   C
   A sore that doesn't heal
   U
   T
   I
   O
   N

A - carrots, peaches, apricots, squash, broccoli

C - grapefruit, cantaloupe, oranges, strawberries

STRESS: PART OF A HEALTHY LIFESTYLE

Stress has a negative connotation in our country, but actually we need some of it. We are confronted with many potential <u>stressors</u> every day. These stressors could be physical, environmental, or psycho-social. Many stressors are positive, or <u>eustress</u>, such as the preparatory arousal for athletic events, spice-of-life kinds of happenings, or the excitement and thrill of other positive, though stressful, events in our lives. Other stressors clearly are <u>distress</u>, such as death in the family, a failing grade, or too much to do in too little time. Some of us operate under too little stress, or <u>hypostress.</u> Others of us operate under too much, or <u>hyperstress</u>. Finding the right amount of stress could be part of a healthy lifestyle.

The physiological stress response is characterized by increased blood pressure, heart rate, cardiac output, plasma free fatty acids, plasma triglycerides, plasma cholesterol, muscle tension, vasoconstriction, and vasodilation. Which of these do you recognize as risk factors for heart disease?

1. The physiological stress above occurs through three different pathways. First, try to recall an event (stressor) in your life that caused a very sudden (split second), powerful stress response. Below, write what the event was, and what you felt physically.

2. Second, some stressors cause a stress response that we can actually feel building up over a short period of time (20 to 30 seconds up to several minutes, for example). Below, write down an event in your life that caused a distinct and noticeable building (as opposed to sudden) of the stress response.

3. Third, some stressors cause a chronic, or long-term stress response. Below, write down an event in your life that you feel caused a great deal of stress over some lengthy period of time, such as days, weeks, or even months. What did you feel, or how could you tell you were under stress?

STRESS PATHWAYS

Short-term Stress Response	Intermediate-term Stress Response	Long-term Stress Response (Chronic)
Sudden, powerful	Builds gradually	Signs vary
Short duration	10X duration	Days, weeks, months
Due to direct end-organ innervation	20-30 second delay, adrenalin secreted into systemic circulation	Endocrine axes: Interaction of endocrine glands

Write two
Write two

Write two

examples below:

examples below:

examples below:

THE TERMINOLOGY OF STRESS

In small groups, define the following terms:

Stressor   Hypostress

Distress   Hyperstress

Eustress   Optimal stress

Types of stressors:	Positive aspects of stress:
Psychological, emotional	Preparatory arousal
Physical (illness, heavy exercise)	Eustress: spice of life
Environmental (heat, cold, noise)	Thrill-seeking, excitement
Social	Maximum effort = self esteem

BUILDING SELF-ESTEEM

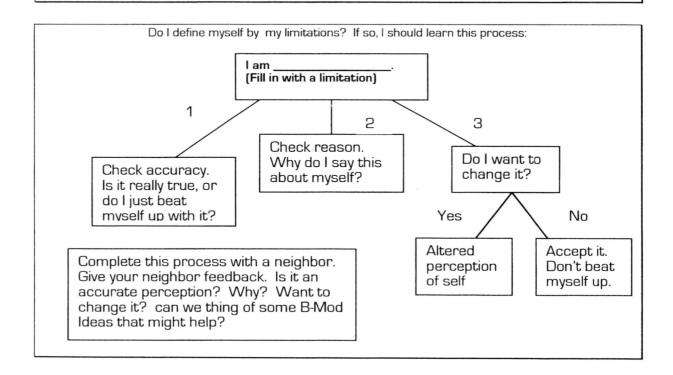

Do I define myself by my limitations? If so, I should learn this process:

I am _____.
(Fill in with a limitation)

1

Check accuracy.
Is it really true, or
do I just beat
myself up with it?

2

Check reason.
Why do I say this
about myself?

3

Do I want to
change it?

Yes

No

Altered
perception
of self

Accept it.
Don't beat
myself up.

Complete this process with a neighbor.
Give your neighbor feedback. Is it an
accurate perception? Why? Want to
change it? can we thing of some B-Mod
Ideas that might help?

THE STRESS RESPONSE

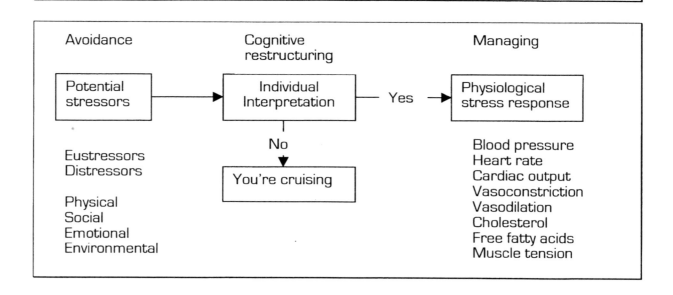

Avoidance

Cognitive
restructuring

Managing

Potential
stressors

Individual
Interpretation

Yes

Physiological
stress response

No

You're cruising

Eustressors
Distressors

Physical
Social
Emotional
Environmental

Blood pressure
Heart rate
Cardiac output
Vasoconstriction
Vasodilation
Cholesterol
Free fatty acids
Muscle tension

INTERRUPTING THE STRESS CYCLE:

THE QR - TRY IT!
DR. JOHN SCHEER

Most of us have, at least occasionally, experienced a high level of stress. We know what the increased heart rate and muscle tension feel like. Other physiological changes take place, as well. For example, our blood pressure, cardiac output, adrenalin, and blood levels of cholesterol, triglycerides and glucose are all increased. For many people who are under chronic stress, these changes can lead to a wide variety of health problems, from heart disease to debilitating back pain.

Obviously, some stress in our lives is desirable. Positive stressors, such as a promotion, pay raise, birth of a child, etc., also cause the physiological stress responses, but these things are the spice of life. We would be pretty bored without some stress. The answer lies in learning to handle stress in a manner that allows us to reduce the physiological changes associated with the stressors we experience.

Research tells us that we need to periodically interrupt the build up of physiological changes that can make the stress response a vicious cycle. A variety of stress management techniques are available. but one that I like, because it is easy and can be used many times every day, is called the Quieting Response (or QR, or 6-second response). Try this:

1. Take a deep breath and raise your shoulders.

2. As you exhale, drop your shoulders.

3. Imagine a wave of warmth flowing out through your arms, hands, and fingers.

4. Make a positive, calming self-statement.

To explain:

1. Stressful breathing is shallow. It is much more relaxing to take deep, abdominal breaths.

2. You can become tuned in to even slight muscle tension. Relaxed muscles are an indication of a relaxed state.

3. Cold, clammy hands are an indication of stress. Warm, dry hands indicate a relaxed state. When we put finger thermometers on students and put them through a stressful task, their finder temperatures often drop into the 70's. We then put them through a relaxation drill, and their finger temperatures often climb into the mid-90's.

4. A positive, calming self-statement can reverse stinking-thinking, which itself can cause the stress response.

Try the QR and practice using it often. Make a habit out of it. You will go a long way toward reversing potentially dangerous build ups of the stress response.

STRESS MANAGEMENT AS A HEALTH
SELF-BEHAVIOR MODIFICATION PROJECT

The following steps, which are consistent with the guiding principles of behavior modification, are effective in helping one to improve the control of stress in his/her life:

1. The log of current behavior, i.e. the collection of baseline information before one starts to change his/her behaviors, would most likely be in the form of a journal.

    a. The log may include the number of times a person feels really stressed.

    b. More importantly, the log should include the kinds of stressors that cause the stress response, what the person feels, and what actions the person takes.

    c. The log should be summarized in a way that clearly and concisely analyzes and describes the stress in a person's life.

2. A reasonable, achievable goal should be established that reflects improvements in stress reduction and management as summarized in the log of current behavior above.

3. The steps that a person can take to go from current behavior to goal behavior are:

    a. Purchase a stress management paperback from a bookstore:
        *Find the section that has stress management paperbacks.
        *Look at the Tables of Contents of a variety of books.
        *When you find a Table of Contents that strikes you as being interesting or has chapter titles that make you want to read it, buy the book.

    b. Read the introductory chapter or two. Most books have chapter(s) that discuss stress in general before going into specific methods of dealing with stress.

    c. Next, read any chapter that you choose. It may be the next chapter, or it may be the chapter that interests you the most.

    d. Borrow one specific idea for reducing stress or for managing stress (two different concepts, by the way!) and use the idea for one week. Write a journal entry every time you use it and whether it works or not. If it works, keep using it and logging it. If it doesn't work, quit using it.

    e. Read another chapter you choose. Use and journal one more idea for a week.

    f. Repeat "d" and "e" above for 8 weeks. At the end of the plan, most people will be regularly using 5 or 6 new stress reduction or management techniques.

4. A reward should be administered every time you complete one of the above steps or use and journal one of the specific techniques for dealing with stress. Good luck!

EFFECTIVE TIME MANAGEMENT:

MAKE SURE YOU'RE GOING SOMEWHERE!

Establishing and prioritizing goals is a necessary step in developing effective time-use skills. Below, list several professional and personal long-term goals and short-term goals you have or would like to have. Prioritize each list as A = high priority; B = medium; C = low priority.

LONG-TERM GOALS [>6 months]   PRIORITY _____

Professional:

Personal:

SHORT-TERM GOALS [< 6 months]   PRIORITY _____

Professional:

Personal:

Now, after you have listed your goals, for seven days make out daily "To Do" lists and prioritize the items. On the "To Do" lists, beside any A priority items you accomplish, jot down the way in which they contribute to the accomplishment of an "A" priority goal you have listed above. Also, circle any "To Do" list item which utilizes the "Swiss Cheese" technique.

HEALTHY LIFESTYLES

FINAL EXAM PREPARATION

The final exam will be 100 multiple choice questions. Bring a calculator and a #2 pencil. Review the course manual, class notes, and textbook Chapters. You should know or be able to do the following:

1. Aerobic exercise effects on the body.

2. How to take EHRs and how to calculate a target zone and use it in an exercise session.

3. Exercise prescription guidelines for frequency, intensity, duration, and mode.

4. Alcohol 0-1-2-4 formula.

5. Food groups and minimum servings, USA averages and government recommendations.

6. Fiber and food labels, average grams per fruit, vegetable, W.G. bread and cereal.

7. Why, how, and when should we stretch?

8. Total, HDL- and LDL- cholesterol; triglycerides; glucose; and follow-up.

9. Self Behavior Modification guiding principles.

10. Role of self-esteem in healthful living, and self-esteem building.

11. Heart disease risk factors and primary risk factors.

12. Effects of strength conditioning on muscle mass, metabolism, and aging.

13. Nutrition math - see study guides in manual.

14. Controlling fat consumption, and reading food labels.

15. Sodium effects and reading food labels.

16. Osteoporosis risk factors, protective factors, and reading food labels.

17. Healthy % fat; calculation of fat, lean, and desirable body weights.

18. Characteristics of good weight loss programs, weight control triangle.

19. Role of exercise in weight control, set point theory (from text), spot reducing.

20. Calculate long-term weight loss from combined exercise and calorie restriction.

21. Short term, intermediate and long-term stress and physiological response.

22. Eustress, distress, and optimal stress. Avoidance, restructuring and managing.

23. Memorize the QR. Try it!

24. Cancer risk factors, protective factors, warning signals, nutraceuticals.

25. Risk factors for AIDS and STDs. HIV testing.

CALCULATING GRADES IN HEALTHY LIFESTYLES

Students frequently want to know exactly how they are doing in the Healthy Lifestyles class. It is important, therefore, to know how the Excel program computes student grades, so that we can give accurate information to students, as well as avoid giving them misinformation.

1. Four factors are graded, and each factor has a percent weighting (a student must pass all four grading factors to pass the course):

   a. Exercise program (lab):   20%
   b. Self Health-Behavior modification project (lab):   20%
   c. Quiz average (class):   20%
   d. Final examination (class):   40%

2. **Exercise program and self heath-behavior modification (lab projects)**. Grades are assigned by consultants to both lab projects. The grades are then converted to grade points and multiplied by the % weighting (20% each):

   A = 4.0; A- = 3.67; B+ = 3.33; B = 3.0; B- = 2.67; C+ = 2.33; C = 2.0;
   C- = 1.67; D+ = 1.33; D = 1.0; D- = 0.67; F = 0.0

3. **Quiz average**. The average percent correct on all quizzes (none are deleted) is converted to grade points according to the chart below, then multiplied by the 20% weighting (Q1% + Q2% + Q3% + Q4%, etc. divided by the number of quizzes).

4. **Final examination**. The score on the 100 item multiple choice final examination is converted to grade points the same way and multiplied by the 40% weighting:

≥94%	= 4.0	81%	= 2.9	70%	= 1.8
92-93%	= 3.9	80%	= 2.8	69%	= 1.7
90-91%	= 3.8	79%	= 2.7	68%	= 1.6
89%	= 3.7	78%	= 2.6	67%	= 1.5
88%	= 3.6	77%	= 2.5	66%	= 1.4
87%	= 3.5	76%	= 2.4	65%	= 1.3
86%	= 3.4	75%	= 2.3	64%	= 1.2
85%	= 3.3	74%	= 2.2	63%	= 1.1
84%	= 3.2	73%	= 2.1	62%	= 1.0
83%	= 3.1	72%	= 2.0	61%	= 0.9
82%	= 3.0	71%	= 1.9	60%	= 0.8	<60% = 0

   The quiz average (using normal rounding) and the final exam score are converted to grade points using the chart above.

5. After multiplying the grade points for each factor by the % weighting, the grade points are totaled and rounded off to the nearest grade (but remember that students must pass all four factors to pass the course):

Excel program computation of final grade:

$\geq$3.84   = A
3.50 – 3.83   = A-
3.17 – 3.49   = B+
2.84 – 3.16   = B
2.50 – 2.83   = B-
2.17 – 2.49   = C+
1.84 – 2.16   = C
1.50 – 1.83   = C-
1.17 – 1.49   = D+
0.84 – 1.16   = D
<1.00   = F

6. Examples:

Student A:	Grade	% Weight	Grade Pts.
Exercise program	A	4.0 x .20	= 0.80
Behavior modification	B	3.0 x .20	= 0.60
Quiz average	76.3%	2.4 x .20	= 0.48
Final examination	66%	1.4 x .40	= 0.56
Accumulated grade points			= 2.44
Final grade			= C+

Student B:	Grade	% Weight	Grade Pts.
Exercise program	A	4.0 x .20	= 0.80
Behavior modification	A	4.0 x .20	= 0.80
Quiz average	88.3%	3.4 x .20	= 0.72
Final examination	91%	3.8 x .40	= 1.52
Accumulated grade points			= 3.84
Final grade			= A

7. Three additional factors can have an impact on a student's grade:

     a. Failure to turn in assignments to lab consultants can result in a reduced grade.
     b. Missing more than one lab results in an automatic F for the course.
     c. If it becomes apparent that lecture attendance is a problem, a reduced grade can be given.